THIS INSPIRING GUIDE EMPOWERS YOU TO TAKE CHARGE OF YOUR HEART HEALTH

A diagnosis of heart disease may be frightening. But the truth is that heart patients can live productive, satisfying lives for years after their diagnosis, and this friendly, accessible guide shows how. Packed with highly useful information, this book tells you everything you need to know to take charge of your heart health, including vital—and potentially lifesaving—information on lifestyle, diet, exercise, medication, surgery, handling emergencies, and finding support groups. Written by one of the country's leading cardiologists and a heart surgery survivor whose own successful battle against a heart problem proves that heart patients can live active, healthy lives, this is a must-have book for all heart patients and their families.

50 ESSENTIAL THINGS TO DO WHEN THE DOCTOR SAYS IT'S HEART DISEASE

DR. FREDRIC J. PASHKOW is the Medical Director of Cardiac Rehabilitation at The Cleveland Clinic Foundation, one of the nation's most prominent cardiology centers. CHARLOTTE LIBOV, an award-winning medical writer, frequently contributes to *The New York Times* and other national publications. A popular speaker on health issues, she lives in Bethlehem, Connecticut. The authors also collaborated on *The Woman's Heart Book* (Dutton/Plume).

50

Essential Things to Do When the Doctor Says It's Heart Disease

Fredric J. Pashkow, M.D.,
and Charlotte Libov

Ⓟ

A PLUME BOOK

PLUME
Published by the Penguin Group
Penguin Books USA Inc., 375 Hudson Street, New York, New York 10014, U.S.A.
Penguin Books Ltd, 27 Wrights Lane, London W8 5TZ, England
Penguin Books Australia Ltd, Ringwood, Victoria, Australia
Penguin Books Canada Ltd, 10 Alcorn Avenue, Toronto, Ontario, Canada M4V 3B2
Penguin Books (N.Z.) Ltd, 182–190 Wairau Road, Auckland 10, New Zealand

Penguin Books Ltd, Registered Offices:
Harmondsworth, Middlesex, England

First published by Plume, an imprint of Dutton Signet,
a division of Penguin Books USA Inc.

First Printing, June, 1995
1 3 5 7 9 10 8 6 4 2

REGISTERED TRADEMARK—MARCA REGISTRADA

LIBRARY OF CONGRESS CATALOGING-IN-PUBLICATION DATA:

Pashkow, Fredric J.
50 essential things to do when the doctor says it's heart disease
/ Fredric J. Pashkow and Charlotte Libov.
p.   cm.
Includes bibliographical references and index.
ISBN 0-452-27101-0
1. Heart—Diseases—Popular works.   I. Libov, Charlotte. II. Title. III. Title: Fifty
essential things to do when the doctor says it's heart disease.
RC672.P37 1995
616.1'2—dc20   94-38921
                                                                 CIP

Printed in the United States of America
Set in Caslon 540 and Caslon Openface

Designed by Steven N. Stathakis

PUBLISHER'S NOTE:
The ideas, procedures and suggestions contained in this book are not intended as a substitute for
consulting with your physician. All matters regarding your health require medical supervision.

Dr. Fredric Pashkow and Charlotte Libov
dedicate this book with love to

Aunt Henny
Uncle Bill
and
Aunt Zelda

CONTENTS

ACKNOWLEDGMENTS

So many people are instrumental over the years in helping an author write a book that it is difficult to acknowledge everyone for their contributions, both large and small. However, for help specifically in preparing this book, the authors would like to thank the following: Holly Atkinson, M.D.; Alan W. Bakst, Pharm.D.; Gordon Blackburn, Ph.D.; Garland Y. DeNelsky, Ph.D.; Israel Gesell, M.S.; Harvey L. Katzeff, M.D.; Richard S. Lang, M.D.; Lynn Luthern, M.A.; Richard N. Matzen, M.D.; Michael G. McGee, Ph.D.; Lynda H. Powell, Ph.D.; Leslie R. Schover, Ph.D.; Wayne Sotile, Ph.D.; and Andrea Vegh Dunn, R.D., L.D.

We also greatly appreciate the research help from the American Heart Association's national office and we offer a special thank-you to Rita Kova Murnane, of the association's Connecticut affiliate. In addition, we wish to thank our editor Deborah Brody, for choosing us to write this book, and Carole Abel, our literary agent, for her support and friendship that goes well beyond her professional role.

Dr. Pashkow wants to thank especially his Cleveland Clinic patients and the readers of *Heartline* whose questions and concerns led to the identification of the "50 Essential Things." For their additional input, Charlotte Libov wants to thank the experts she interviewed and the patients who shared their stories. On a personal note, she also wants to thank her other family members, particularly Aunt Evelyn and Uncle Jerry, for their unwavering support, and, of course Terry Montlick, for his contributions in ways too numerous to mention.

PART ONE

ESSENTIAL UNDERSTANDING

CHAPTER ONE

INTRODUCTION:
HEART DISEASE
AND YOU

Heart disease is the number one killer of American men and women. There's no disputing that fact. The purpose of this book, however, is not to dwell on the negative. Today, millions of people with heart disease enjoy active, satisfying lives. Their secret? Instead of looking upon a diagnosis of heart disease as a sentence to be a "cardiac invalid" for life, they have used their diagnosis of heart disease to their advantage. They've used it as a catalyst, an event which propelled them to make positive changes in their life. This book is intended to help you become one of them.

When doctors first began studying atherosclerosis, the process by which coronary arteries become narrowed, they believed it was irreversible. Over the years, this has been found untrue. By making changes in your lifestyle, obtaining the correct medical care, and using your mind to help your body, you can "beat" heart disease. This does not mean that your arteries will be transformed from narrow and clogged to squeaky clean, or that heart muscle damaged by a heart attack will be rejuvenated. It *does* mean that heart disease can be turned into a positive force in your life.

Consider Ken. A small-town pharmacist, Ken was only thirty-nine when he learned he had a heart problem. Although heart disease ran in his family, Ken did not dream he had a heart problem until one day, when he was exercising at a local gym. "I suddenly realized something was wrong," he said. He felt sweaty and faint. He had severe pressure in the center of his chest. His pulse was irregular. The diagnosis? Heart disease.

Now, nearly three years after his diagnosis, Ken feels fine. True, his life is not exactly the way it was before. He underwent a balloon angioplasty procedure, he watches his diet, and he takes medication to lower his cholesterol.

In many ways, though, Ken finds his life is better. He's more aware of when he is under stress. He takes customary days off. He exercises regularly instead of just "fitting it in." "Before, I didn't think of my health, and I was apt to burn the candle at both ends. Now, I take care of myself and that's made a big difference," he says.

Linda, a fifty-eight-year-old nurse, did not discover she had heart disease until she suffered a heart attack. At the time, she smoked heavily. Now, she's given up cigarettes. She's also given up the junk food in (of all places!) the nurses' lounge. Instead of just telling her patients to eat right and exercise, she's joined them! She looks, and feels, ten years younger.

If you have coronary artery disease, by making the lifestyle changes outlined in this book, such as quitting smoking, reducing dietary fat, and participating in regular physical exercise, you may be able to slow or even stop the development of the hard fatty material that is clogging your arteries. In that way, you are "beating" heart disease.

If you have more severe heart disease, or if your heart was damaged by a heart attack, you won't be able to do the same things that someone in perfect physical shape can do: You may tire easily and have to restrict your physical activity. But, working with your doctor, you can create a satisfying way of life. Perhaps you'll have to give up mountain climbing, but hiking may still be open to you. You may be surprised at how much pleasure life still holds for you.

THE "KNOW-YOUR-HEART" ESSENTIALS

Knowledge is your key to dealing with heart disease. So, before getting started on our 50 "Essentials," it's important to understand how your heart works.

The human body is truly amazing. Biologically, we are comprised of a collection of organs which work in unison, creating the processes which keep us functioning perfectly. Of all those organs, none is more miraculous than the heart. Breathtaking in its simplicity, the heart is awe-inspiring when you consider its tremendous workload. Your heart keeps about five quarts of blood circulating through a pathway of blood vessels that would measure approximately seventy-five thousand miles if laid end-to-end. And it does so, without a pause, for your entire life.

Your circulatory system includes your heart, lungs, arteries and capillaries (extremely small blood vessels), as well as your veins, through which blood flows on its return to the heart. Men and women's circulatory systems are essentially the same, though the components of a woman's are slightly smaller.

The basic job of your heart is to pump blood. Actually, your heart contains two pumps which act separately but in concert. The left side of your heart acts as a high-pressure pump which forces oxygen-rich blood out into all the parts of your body. The right side of your heart receives the oxygen-depleted blood and passes it into the lungs, where it is replenished with oxygen. The blood then flows into the left side of the heart, to begin its journey again.

Your heart's primary role is to pump oxygen-rich blood to feed every cell in your body, and then pump the unoxygenated blood out to the lungs again. This furnishes your organs with the oxygen they need. But your heart also needs oxygen-rich blood to live. Furnishing your heart with this needed oxygen is the job of your three coronary arteries, which lie on the surface of your heart. They are shaped like the winding tubes of the musical instrument the coronet, hence the name, "coronary" arteries.

Your heart also has its own electrical system, which stimulates it to contract an average of 100,000 times per day. Each heartbeat originates in a specific area of the right atrium called the sino-atrial node. This is often referred to as your heart's intrinsic pacemaker. If anything goes wrong with this electrical system, such as damage from a heart attack, the result can be an irregular heartbeat, also known as an arrhythmia. Arrhythmias are often treated with drug therapy.

As the blood makes its journey through the heart, it's very important that it flow only in one direction. Four heart valves ensure this proper flow and see to it that blood which is filled with oxygen does not get mixed with unoxygenated blood.

Even with heart disease, your heart remains a miraculous organ capable of performing its magnificent job. But since heart disease can make that job more difficult, it's up to you to make your heart's work easier, so it can continue to pump away for many, many years to come.

What You Can Do: Explore your local library, your local affiliate of the American Heart Association, or the "Resources" section of this book, to find more information about how your heart works. The more understanding you have, the more knowledgeable and motivated you'll be to undertake the "essential" steps to conquer heart disease.

HEART DISEASE: "RISKY BUSINESS"

When Harry had his heart attack, there seemed to be no question why. Harry was a smoker, stuffed himself with bacon and eggs at every opportunity, and regularly proclaimed, in a loud voice, "I'm 'allergic' to exercise!"

There are 6.2 million Americans currently living with heart disease. Experts estimate that in about 50 percent of the cases, risk factors, such as those exemplified by Harry, contributed to their cause.

Most often when risk factors are discussed, they are considered in the context of heart disease prevention. So discussing risk factors now, after you've been diagnosed with heart disease, may seem like shutting the barn door after the horse has fled. But this is not really the case. When risk factors are discussed as a means of preventing heart disease, it's called "primary prevention." But working to modify risk factors now can be beneficial as well. Technically, this is known as "secondary" prevention. But we don't consider it "secondary" at all, and neither should you. After all, when you have heart disease, working to minimize risk factors can mean the difference between life and death. By reducing your risks, you may reduce the probability you will suffer a heart attack or require coronary bypass surgery.

The major risk factors for heart disease are:

- Smoking.
- A family history of heart disease. In other words, a primary relative (father, mother, sister, brother) who suffered a heart attack or developed coronary artery disease before the age of fifty-five.
- High blood cholesterol levels.

- Poorly controlled diabetes with high blood-sugar levels.
- Uncontrolled high blood pressure.
- Being male or a female past menopause.
- Lack of exercise.
- Stress. Most experts agree it plays at least a contributing role. For more on stress, see chapter 8.

Reducing risk factors is made all the easier because they are often interconnected. For example, if you are overweight, losing weight may help bring down your blood cholesterol level. Exercising not only helps weight loss but lessens stress, decreases high blood pressure, and helps control diabetes.

Throughout this book, we'll show you "essential" ways to reduce your heart disease risk, and put the odds in your favor.

What You Can Do: On a piece of paper, evaluate your risk factors for heart disease. Consider the ones that you can change. For example, if you have diabetes, it will not disappear. But, by exercising, you can bring it under better control. What other risk factors can you change?

Essentials (For Women Only)

This is not one of those heart-care books which relegates women to a less important role. All of the recommendations in this book, except where specifically noted, apply to both women and men. However, because heart disease in females has been dangerously overlooked, women need to keep some particular points in mind to make certain they are getting the best possible care for their hearts.

Traditionally, heart disease was viewed as a man's health problem. Early studies suggested that heart disease occurred almost solely in men, while women were viewed as virtually immune. Today, we know that to be false. For most of this century, heart disease has been the number one cause of death among both women and men.

It is also important to recognize that virtually all of the research on heart disease has been done on men. There have been a few large-scale studies done on women, but these are the exception. Most traditional methods of diagnosing and treating heart disease appear to be effective in both men and women, but they were developed almost solely using men. So, for your own tests and treatments, ask your doctor about special considerations for women.

The big difference between heart disease in men and women is age. Up until menopause, women generally do not develop heart disease. The qualification "generally" is very important. It's true most of the time, but sometimes a younger woman may develop heart disease, especially if she has a major risk factor such as diabetes.

Although it was assumed that risk factors in men and in women were the same, researchers are now finding subtle, but important, differences. For example, a fifty-five-year-old woman who smokes, who has elevated cholesterol and high blood pressure, has three times the normal risk for a heart attack. In comparison, a fifty-five-year-old man with exactly the same risk factors has only double the normal risk. Taking oral contraceptives by themselves is generally not a risk but, combined with smoking, becomes a major heart attack risk factor.

As a woman, you need to be aware of an issue known as "gender bias." This term refers to studies that have shown that women with heart disease are treated differently than men. The studies showed men were twice as likely to undergo cardiac catheterization, the common diagnostic procedure a patient must have before undergoing such treatments as balloon angioplasty and coronary bypass surgery. Is this necessarily bad? Perhaps. But, on the other hand, research also indicates that these "aggressive" treatments may be overused.

There are certain societal factors which may also affect a woman's heart. Women tend to fare worse after a heart attack, partly because women are usually older than men when first afflicted. But studies have also shown women with heart problems tend to suffer from depression more. They are also more likely to be socially isolated or to lack good health insurance. Furthermore, studies show that women tend to delay treatment and more often refuse to be transferred from community hospitals to larger institutions that offer more sophisticated care.

Make certain that your complaints are taken seriously, your symptoms thoroughly evaluated and you are not overlooked for certain treatments simply because you are a woman. Ask questions. Do your homework. Since women sometimes face more complications from treatments such as balloon angioplasty and coronary bypass surgery, choose your doctor and hospital with care if you need these treatments. Enlist your family as your support team. You can put the odds in your favor.

PART TWO

The 50 Essential Things to Do

CHAPTER TWO

GETTING STARTED

We believe very strongly in all of the 50 essential things we outline in this book. Patients have found these steps very useful and, in some instances, lifesaving. There are, however, some very important steps you need to take now to start creating your own plan to combat heart disease. This chapter describes these crucial first steps.

#1

Empower Yourself

Back in the old days, when you went to a doctor, you expected that you would be taken care of. This implied that you, as patient, were a passive vessel, similar to a car brought into the service shop for repair. The responsibility for returning you to a state of normal health, i.e. "good running order," was entirely up to your doctor.

How times have changed! Today, your doctor is more your coach than your mechanic. He or she is there to provide you with expertise and guidance. But you're the one with the ultimate responsibility to get things going right.

What happened? How did we go so quickly from a state of total dependency to one of self-responsibility?

From the doctor's perspective, it probably started with the so-called malpractice problem. As the threat of malpractice actions grew during the 1970s, it occurred to most doctors that many illnesses and injuries were, in fact, at least partially self-inflicted. Sometimes the patient had failed to do what could have been done to achieve optimal recovery and return to health.

For example, consider Walter, a sixty-six-year-old who resumed cigarette smoking after undergoing coronary bypass surgery. Such smoking can lead to a "premature" failure of the procedure; that is, the grafts that were created to provide an alternate flow of blood to the heart close more quickly than in someone who chose to quit.

So, whose "fault" was it when Walter returned with symptoms in a few months? Did the surgeon "screw up" or did the accumulated poisons from the two packs of cigarettes per day that Walter couldn't live without cause the problem?

In most of these cases, we may never really know. But it is at least possible that Walter was partly responsible.

Things have changed from the patient's perspective as well. Over two decades ago, Ralph Nader helped usher in an "age of consumerism." People began to question aspects of their lives which they previously had taken for granted. This occurred in all facets of daily life—government, schools, and medicine as well.

So patients and doctors began expecting more of each other. We think this is all to the good. Patients should not be viewed as passive vessels, nor doctors as God.

Imagine yourself as Walter. If you were ordered to simply stop smoking but given no specific reasons, you might be less inclined to stop. If, however, you were provided with information about how smoking directly affects your bypass graft, as well as provided with information and support to help you quit, your chance of success would be greatly increased.

"Empowerment" is the new buzzword for this concept. Your doctor is responsible for doing his or her best on your behalf, but you have the responsibility for doing all you can to positively affect your own health.

That's what this book is all about. It places in your

hands 50 steps you can take, right now, to help your heart. By taking action, you empower yourself.

> *What You Can Do:* Start thinking in a proactive manner. Learn what you can do about your problem. What options do you have? What steps can you take to make your therapy a success?

#2

Learn the Lingo

To deal effectively with heart disease, you need to know the language. Dealing with heart disease, or any serious illness, for that matter, is a bit like being suddenly deposited in a foreign country. In a foreign land, most of us feel most comfortable if we can at least ask the basics, like where the bathroom is, and how much the bus costs.

Cardiology, the "land of the heart," is not much different. You'll want to be able to communicate with the "natives" (the doctors, nurses, and lab technicians) effectively. By speaking the same language, you'll be empowered. You'll be less likely to be intimidated, and you can better absorb information from the media.

Cardiac means pertaining to the heart; hence, *cardiology* is the study of the heart, and a *cardiologist* is a doctor who specializes in the study and treatment of the heart. (Note: Doctors tend to refer to almost all heart problems by using the umbrella term "heart disease." They use the term when speaking of congenital heart defects, which are heart problems people are born with, heart valve problems, or irregular heartbeats. But when most people use the term "heart disease" what they are really talking about is *coronary heart disease*. In this book, we use the terms "heart disease" and "coronary heart disease" interchangeably. But, unless we specify otherwise, we always mean coronary heart disease.)

Coronary heart disease is a particular type of heart disease, the one most people talk about when they refer to atherosclerosis, a buildup of fatty material in the artery wall which causes it to become thickened and irregular. This buildup, sometimes called *plaque*, results in a narrowing of the coronary arteries.

Studies have also shown that, by making lifestyle changes, such as those outlined in this book regarding eating, exercise, and quitting smoking, you may be able to accomplish a *regression* in the process of atherosclerosis. In fact, studies show that making heart-healthy lifestyle changes can result in a 5 to 10 percent regression of atherosclerosis. That may not sound like much, but it could mean the difference between having a heart attack or requiring coronary bypass surgery and avoiding it.

Blood carries oxygen to all the tissues of the body including your heart, which needs oxygen to survive. If this oxygen is cut off, this can result in a *heart attack*, permanent damage to the heart muscle caused by a lack of blood supply to the heart for an extended period.

There are different ways to diagnose heart disease. You may have already undergone some of these tests. An *electrocardiogram*, known also as an EKG (or ECG), is the familiar test in which electrodes are placed on your chest and a picture of your heartbeat is conveyed on graph paper. This picture shows the electrical impulses traveling through the heart muscle. An *exercise (EKG) "stress test"* is a diagnostic procedure in which an activity, such as walking on a treadmill or riding a stationary bicycle, is used to evaluate the effect of physical exertion on the heart.

Another diagnostic test, an *echocardiogram*, uses ultrasound to detect and electronically record structural and some functional abnormalities of the heart, like a malfunctioning heart valve. Although traditionally an echocardiogram is not used to diagnose coronary artery disease, it can be a useful tool if combined with an exercise stress test. This is sometimes called an *"exercise echo."*

All these tests we've described are *noninvasive*, which means they don't require any instruments to penetrate the body, and are generally painless and nearly risk-free. Such tests can indicate you have heart disease, but do not completely evaluate its extent. Your doctor may then turn to what has been termed the "gold standard" of cardiac testing, *cardiac catheterization*, known also as *coronary angiography*. In this procedure, a tube is inserted into an artery in the arm or leg and guided to the heart. Contrast dye is injected and X-ray movies are taken of the dye flowing through the coronary arteries. The progression of the dye gauges the extent of the narrowing of the arteries. Thus, your doctor is provided with a "road map" of your coronary arteries that pinpoints exactly where any narrowing or blockages are. This test is required before such procedures as coronary bypass surgery and balloon angioplasty.

Coronary artery disease can be treated in a variety of ways. *Cardiovascular drugs*, for example, can be used to lower high blood pressure, reduce cholesterol, and to ease the symptoms of heart disease.

There is another class of drugs which are administered during a heart attack to abort the attack itself. These are called *thrombolytic* drugs, or *"clot busters."* If used in time, they can dissolve the blood clot that caused the heart attack and minimize the amount of damage to the heart muscle that the attack could cause.

The main surgical treatment for coronary artery disease is *coronary bypass surgery*. Pioneered in the 1960s, this very common procedure involves taking a vein from the leg or artery from the chest and using it as a conduit (a "pipe") to bypass the blockage and create an alternate flow of blood to the heart.

More recently, however, an alternative treatment that does not require opening the chest has gained great popularity. This is *balloon angioplasty*, a procedure used to widen narrowed arteries. Unlike coronary bypass surgery, no new conduit is created. Instead, a balloon-tipped catheter is passed into the narrowed segment of the artery from an entry point in the groin. The balloon is inflated and the artery opened (or dilated). There are related procedures, such as *atherectomy*, in which tiny drill-like or bladelike instruments drill through or shave the atherosclerotic plaque causing the narrowing.

If you've experienced a heart attack, or undergone coronary bypass surgery or balloon angioplasty, you may have been referred for *cardiac rehabilitation*. This program of exercise, psychological and social support is designed to return people to normalcy or better after a heart attack or other cardiac crisis. It can be used as a treatment for heart disease alone, or following coronary bypass surgery, angioplasty, or atherectomy.

Throughout this book, we will return to these terms and go into some of them in more depth. There will be others to learn as we go along. As with any other experience, it's always easier to talk with professionals if you "know the language."

What You Can Do: Learn and practice the terminology of cardiology by clipping an article about heart disease from a newspaper or magazine or read a book on the subject. If some terms are not clear, look them up in a medical dictionary or discuss them with your doctor or other health professional. Never hesitate to ask questions.

#3

Choose the Right Doctor

If you have a solid, longtime relationship with your cardiologist, you may be tempted to skip this section. Don't. At some point, your cardiologist may retire. Or you may find yourself joining a health maintenance organization (HMO), or some other type of system. Or you may outlive your physician!

On the other hand, you may be uncertain that your current cardiologist is best for you. Perhaps you did not know you had heart disease, but, upon suffering a heart attack, you were assigned a cardiologist at the hospital. No matter what the circumstances, since the doctor is the captain of your team, it is very important that he or she be top-notch. Do your homework. Choosing the right doctor may turn out to be one of the most important decisions you'll make. How long you'll live and the quality of your life may depend on it.

We are often asked, "How important is a doctor's personality?" That's hard to say. Skill should be your paramount concern. But if you are constantly at odds with your doctor, if you feel patronized, or uneasy for any reason, this is reason enough to consider finding someone new.

We're also often asked if women should specifically seek out a female doctor. Because of the growing number of women cardiologists, this is becoming an option. We don't believe male cardiologists should be automatically excluded because of their gender. There are a lot of very skilled, sensitive male doctors in practice. However, if you'd prefer a female doctor, you should feel free to seek one.

Choose a doctor who communicates well. Two-way communication is an essential part of keeping you healthy. You should never be made to feel stupid when you ask a question, no matter what it is. It's important to feel comfortable when you ask questions, and you should be answered in terms you can understand.

Your cardiologist should make you feel that your visit and your problems are the major focus of his or her attention. During your visit, you should be made to feel that your well-being is the most important factor in the world.

When you choose a doctor, you are also often choosing a hospital. Doctors have "privileges." This means they are only permitted to practice in certain hospitals. If you need hospitalization, you will be admitted where your doctor practices. If you like the doctor, but you have reservations about the hospital where he or she works, that's a consideration. See our section on "Choose the Right Hospital" (page 78).

Trust your gut feelings. Sometimes, you may distrust a doctor for no particular reason, but some undefinable "something" makes you feel uneasy. If that is the case, you probably won't be able to build the type of doctor-patient relationship you need. Try someone else. Remember, though, that doctors are not infallible. Don't "doctor shop" without cause.

What You Can Do: If you are choosing a new cardiologist (or other type of doctor), here are some essential steps:

- Call your local medical society or American Heart Association affiliate and ask for a directory or referral guide. This lists the education, training, and sometimes the special interests of the doctors in your area.
- Check the doctor's background. Look for degrees and documentation of training from the best medical schools and institutions. While this is no guarantee, it can be an indication of quality.
- Ask the right people. If you have friends who are health professionals, ask who they go to and why. Hospital nurses have an excellent vantage point for seeing doctors in action.

#4

MAKE THE MOST OF DOCTOR'S VISITS

Too often, we await our visits with our doctors with anticipation, only to discover afterward that we've forgotten to ask about the most important thing that was bothering us. In order to have an effective relationship with your doctor, you need to make every visit count. Here are tips on getting the most out of your doctor's visits:

- Keep your doctor informed. For example, if you have heart disease, you may very well suffer from angina. Tell your doctor if you experience more frequent or intense chest pain, or such symptoms as shortness of breath or bodily swelling. Too often, patients are tempted to keep such information to themselves out of fear or worry.
- Respect your doctor's time. Your doctor should respect your time, and you, in turn, should respect his or hers. Your doctor should not hurry you out of the office, but you should realize your doctor's time is limited as well. If you want

your doctor's undivided attention to discuss a new, complicated course of treatment or lifestyle change, consider
scheduling an extra appointment. This may be well worth
the extra fee.

- If you are interested in getting your doctor's opinion on
health news of interest, bring along the clippings. Resist
the temptation to immediately call your doctor every time
you find something of interest, unless you see something
which seems very important, like a warning issued on a
drug you are taking.

- Be pleasant. Remember, your doctor may be having a
stressful day as well. If your doctor is continually rude or insensitive, consider another doctor. But an uncharacteristic-
ally insensitive remark may signify nothing more than your
doctor is having a bad day.

- Consider your doctor to be responsible for your medical
care, but don't blame him or her for events outside their
control. Sometimes, a course of treatment may fail despite
everyone's best effort.

What You Can Do:

- Before your doctor's appointment, write down a
list of your concerns and carry it into the office
with you. Put them in priority; if you don't cover
them all, ask your doctor if you can call or make
a follow-up visit to discuss the rest. Take a list of
your medications, too.

- Consider taking a family member or friend along
with you to act as a "listener." It is sometimes impossible to absorb all the medical news about
your condition and you might find that after
you've left the doctor's office you've forgotten
valuable information.

- Certainly ask questions, but don't have a full discussion of your health concerns while you are still undressed. As Holly Atkinson, M.D., notes, it's impossible to feel empowered when you're sitting on an examining table almost naked.

#5

GET SECOND OPINIONS
(WHEN NEEDED)

There may be several options and no clear-cut correct course for treating heart disease. So, the time may come when you may wonder if a recommendation for, say, balloon angioplasty or coronary bypass surgery is the wisest alternative. Or, you may want to know more about your options.

For example, after learning that she had heart disease, Grace was confronted with three choices and told she must decide quickly. "I was told I could be treated with drugs, balloon angioplasty, or bypass surgery." She was not given much information about the pros or cons of the three procedures, and she opted for the bypass surgery. Now, she's having second thoughts. "Maybe I didn't need to subject myself to the surgery. I'll always wonder if I made the right choice," she says.

Getting a second opinion can sometimes be a lifesaver. After Joe suffered a heart attack in England, his doctor said nothing could be done. Joe's family sought out another doctor, who recommended a coronary bypass. He's doing well today.

Here are some examples of when you might seek a second opinion. Keep in mind that these are only examples; the possible situations are almost endless.

Consider seeking a second opinion if, for example:

- You are concerned about symptoms which seem cardiac-related, but your doctor brushes off your concerns.
- You're taking cardiovascular drugs, but your symptoms are getting worse, and your doctor is not inclined to investigate further.
- You've been told you need open-heart surgery, but you are considered too old to survive it.
- You've been told coronary bypass surgery is your best route, but you wonder if the possibility of a less invasive procedure, such as balloon angioplasty, has been fully explored.

How should you find a doctor to give you that second opinion? Some people believe that doctors tend to stick together, so someone recommended by your doctor is likely to be only a "rubber stamp." Others disagree. They contend that, since your doctor knows your medical problem best, asking that physician for a recommendation is only logical. Listen to your gut. If you are confident your doctor's recommendation will be objective, do so. If you are uncertain, follow our steps for choosing a cardiologist (see step 3, page 22).

So what if you got that second opinion and it's the opposite of the first? Experts can disagree. Since your heart's health is at stake, you may have to seek out a third opinion to be the tie-breaker. With three opinions, it's time to make a decision. Seeking a second opinion (or even a third) if you are in a situation which calls for one is one of the most essential things you can do to safeguard your well-being.

What You Can Do:
- Check your health insurance policy. In the case of many cardiac procedures, second opinions are not optional, they're required.
- In the midst of a health crisis, it may seem like too much trouble to begin doing the homework necessary to find the right doctor to offer a second opinion. Talk to a relative or close friend; they may be able to do this research on your behalf.

#6

Quit Smoking

In this book, we offer you 50 essential steps to take if you have heart disease. Some are optional. Smoking isn't. Quitting is absolutely essential. Let the other forty-nine slide for now if you want. That's how strongly we feel about this.

Here are the facts:

Each time you inhale cigarette smoke, you are breathing a mixture of four thousand chemical substances—many of them poisonous—into your body. When you inhale cigarette smoke, sulfuric acid not only eats away at the tissue of your lungs, but damages the blood vessels of your heart as well. Studies have shown smoking can also adversely affect your cholesterol levels. And smoking, by the way, is an equal opportunity killer, deadly to both men and women.

But, as you'd probably be the first to tell us, quitting smoking isn't that easy. This is because smoking is often a complicated physical and emotional addiction, notes Garland Y. DeNelsky, Ph.D., an expert on smoking at the Cleveland Clinic's Department of Psychiatry and Psychology.

First and foremost, he notes, smoking is a physical addiction. The extent of this addiction can vary: Some people remain virtually nonaddicted and can easily give up smoking. But, for most people, smoking is a powerful physical addiction, similar to such strong addictions as heroin and cocaine.

Second, smoking is an ingrained behavioral pattern. People smoke in certain situations, frequently in response to certain stimuli. These situations quickly become linked in the smoker's mind with the act of smoking.

For example, when Lynn gave up smoking eight years ago, she also gave up coffee. "Even the smell of coffee would make me yearn for a cigarette," recalls Lynn, who now sticks to tea.

Smoking often takes on a personal, psychological meaning to the smoker. For some, a cigarette may become a "best friend," or an impossible-to-substitute way of handling stress. Smoking can seem to be a necessity, both in happy and unhappy situations, notes Dr. DeNelsky. "When a smoker gets a raise, he lights a cigarette to celebrate." But when that same smoker smashes the front fender of his car, he also turns to a cigarette, this time to ease the pain.

Women, especially, tend to look to cigarettes both as a means of handling stress and as a way of keeping their weight down. This is a tempting, but shortsighted practice.

Since smoking is a form of addiction, 80 percent of smokers who quit usually experience some form of withdrawal symptoms. These symptoms may be intense for two or three days, but within ten to fourteen days after quitting, most subside. Interestingly, studies show the 20 percent who do not report withdrawal symptoms are often heart attack survivors. Sometimes, suffering a heart attack, or being diagnosed with heart disease, is enough incentive to quit. Unfortunately, though, often it is not.

What's the most successful way to quit? According to Dr. DeNelsky, studies show that 85 to 90 percent of people who actually quit do so on their own. Also, like Lynn, they seem to develop their own, individualized coping strategies. But for some people, especially those who have been unsuccessful on their own, some type of smoking cessation program can be useful. Lynn, for example, used a free guide from the American Lung Association called "Freedom from Smoking in 20 Days."

Whether you design your own plan or join an established program, it is essential to figure out what works for you. If quitting smoking brings on withdrawal symptoms, consider a nicotine substitute, such as the popular patch system. Research shows, though, that the patch is mainly effective when combined with participation in a smoking cessation program. Also, since the patch delivers nicotine directly into your body, you should use these only under the direction of your doctor. If you smoke with the patch on, you're getting a dangerous double dose of nicotine, which could cause serious cardiac problems, such as angina or even a heart attack.

The essential thing about quitting smoking is to do it. Sometimes, it will take several tries. But keep the faith. Remember, millions of people have quit and you can be one of them. The risk of smoking is great, but the odds of quitting are on your side.

What You Can Do:
- Set your resolve. You may have tried before, but this time you'll make it.
- Ask your local chapters of the American Heart Association, the American Cancer Society, and the American Lung Association for free materials on how to quit smoking.

- Reward yourself for your success! Take the money you spent on cigarettes and put it aside. Buy yourself something special or pamper yourself with a day at a spa. You deserve it!

HELP YOUR LOVED
ONE(S) QUIT, TOO

If your spouse, sibling, offspring, or someone else who shares your home smokes, urge them to quit. Long suspected as harmful, so-called "passive" or "secondhand" smoke is now considered a Group A, or known human carcinogen, by the federal Environmental Protection Agency. This puts it in the same category as such dangerous cancer-causing substances as asbestos.

Infants and young children whose parents smoke are among the most seriously affected by exposure to secondhand smoke, being at increased risk of lower respiratory infections such as pneumonia and bronchitis. Asthmatic children are also at risk.

But adults are also harmed by secondhand smoke, experts say. Numerous studies, which typically looked at non-smoking wives and their exposure to their husband's cigarette smoking, has found exposure to this tobacco smoke harmful. Health experts blame passive smoke for the deaths of up to forty thousand nonsmokers annually. That's nearly the number of women who die each year from breast cancer!

In the previous section, we enumerated the ways that smoking damages your heart. Since that damage can come from the tobacco smoke you inhale voluntarily, or from someone else's cigarette, it is imperative that you not be exposed to cigarette smoke. Obviously, you should not become a prisoner in your smoke-free house. But you should make every effort to discourage public smoking.

What You Can Do:
- If your loved ones have tried to quit before, don't remind them of past failures. Be positive.
- Be encouraging, not a nag. If cigarettes are a continual point of conflict between you and your spouse, consider that the issue may be more than just smoking.
- Fight passive smoke by working with your local government to enact smoking bans in public places such as restaurants, government buildings, and the workplace. Be sympathetic to the plight of smokers, 70 percent of whom would elect to quit if they could, but be firm! Smoking is not appropriate in public places or in the work environment.

#8

LOWER YOUR HIGH
BLOOD PRESSURE

Heart disease and high blood pressure often go together. If you have both of these conditions, it is very important to control your blood pressure because if untreated, high blood pressure can lead to a worsening of your heart disease or eventually a stroke.

Understanding how high blood pressure damages your heart can better motivate you to control it. Longstanding high blood pressure results in what is called hypertensive cardiovascular disease, a condition in which your heart muscle thickens and the heart eventually weakens. While most people are screened for high blood pressure, this disease is still quite common.

High blood pressure also contributes to atherosclerosis, the buildup of fat-containing deposits within your arteries, which often narrow them, resulting in coronary artery disease. To envision how this happens, think of your circulatory system as a river. At some places, where the river is narrow, pressure can build up and create turbulence, which can erode the banks of the river.

The same thing can occur within your body. If your coronary arteries have been narrowed by heart disease, blood pressure can build. This high pressure can damage the walls of your arteries. As your body attempts to repair the damage, further narrowing can result. As if this was not bad enough, high blood pressure increases the workload on your heart, causing a greater demand for oxygen. So, if you have narrowed coronary arteries, or a heart damaged by a heart attack, high blood pressure can be very dangerous indeed.

If you have borderline high blood pressure, your doctor may advise you to control it by losing weight, exercising, quitting smoking, and cutting down on salt if you are "salt sensitive" (to find out if you are, read on). If you have severe hypertension, these steps, plus medication, will be prescribed. Some types of medication are useful in both the control of coronary heart disease and high blood pressure. Reducing stress can also be beneficial.

Some people who have high blood pressure are sensitive to salt, but others are not. For some, sodium (salt) causes fluid retention, which puts an added burden on the heart. Try eliminating salt; if it turns out you are not salt sensitive, you don't need to avoid it.

You should also watch your alcohol intake: Heavy drinking can make blood pressure rise. If you experience adverse effects from high blood pressure medications, don't discontinue them; discuss it with your doctor. A change in medication or schedule may solve the problem. Don't be discouraged if you must continue medication indefinitely. Remember the treatment is far less than what is required to treat the deadly complications of untreated high blood pressure.

Regular aerobic exercise, even brisk walking, can pay big dividends. Just ask Evelyn. Many years ago, she developed high blood pressure. After experiencing a back problem, she decided to ask her doctor about exercise to increase her fitness. She soon began a walking program, and was delighted to find her blood pressure dropped so much her doctor was able to decrease her medication! "I wish I'd known about walking years ago. I would have been happy to do it all these years," says Evelyn.

Whether or not you *develop* high blood pressure may be impossible for you to control. However, what you *can* control is your blood pressure level. Keeping it under control minimizes the chance that it will damage your heart.

What You Can Do:
- Learn to take your blood pressure at home with reliable equipment. Your local affiliate of the American Heart Association has brochures filled with tips on lowering high blood pressure and on buying home blood pressure equipment. Keep regular records of your blood pressure. Your doctor can use this information in determining your correct medication.

What Is High Blood Pressure?

Category	Systolic [upper number] (mmHg)	Diastolic [lower number] (mmHg)
Normal Blood Pressure	Less than 130	Less than 85
High normal	130–139	85–89
High Blood Pressure		
Stage 1 (mild)	140–159	90–99
Stage 2 (moderate)	160–179	100–109
Stage 3 (severe)	180–209	110–119
Stage 4 (very severe)	210 or higher	120 or higher

Source: *Heartline*

Control Your Diabetes

Like heart disease, diabetes and high blood pressure commonly go together. If you have both, you are at much greater risk of suffering a heart attack, especially if you are a woman. However, no matter whether you are male or female, you are at increased risk, and there are some steps you should take to minimize it.

Diabetics are at increased risk of being unaware of an important warning sign of a heart attack: chest pain. Diabetes causes a type of nerve damage called neuropathy, which can interfere with your brain's normal perception of pain. Because of this, you may perceive pain in your chest that is unrelated to heart disease. On the other hand, you may not feel any pain at all when in fact your body is trying to signal you that a heart attack is imminent. As Dr. Harvey L. Katzeff, a diabetes researcher with the Cornell University Medical College notes, "people with diabetes really cannot trust their own instincts."

This is what happened to Harry, a sixty-five-year-old diabetic. One night, he felt pain in his shoulder and arm. A builder, he figured he'd hurt himself on the job, although he really didn't recall any injury. He took some aspirin, but the sensation did not go away. By the time he finally got to the hospital, his heart had been severely damaged.

Myrna, a fifty-six-year-old woman, was also diabetic, but unaware she suffered from heart disease. She was feeling poorly, but figured she had the flu. Tests showed she actually had congestive heart failure. Her heart had been damaged by a heart attack of which Myrna had been unaware.

To keep on top of your condition, your cardiologist should monitor you closely and have you undergo cardiac tests every year or so to evaluate the extent of your heart disease. Tests such as exercise stress tests are more difficult to administer in diabetics because of fluctuations in blood sugar levels, so be certain your test is done in a hospital or laboratory accustomed to testing diabetics.

If you have both diabetes and heart disease, you may find yourself seeing more than one doctor, such as a primary care physician (or internist or family doctor), and a cardiologist. Make sure that any doctor you see is aware that you have both diabetes *and* heart disease. Some cardiovascular medications and cholesterol-lowering medications can interfere with blood sugar control. Be aware of such potential medication interactions.

If you smoke, you must quit. Diabetics are prone to "peripheral vascular disease," a narrowing of the arteries which can lead to a heart attack. Nicotine is a vasoconstrictor that induces this type of vascular narrowing. So, smoking is particularly deadly for diabetics.

Studies have shown that diabetics who undertake a daily program of thirty to forty minutes of aerobic exercise significantly reduce their risk of a heart attack. The advantages of exercise are particularly important if, like many heart disease patients, you have this dangerous trio: heart disease, high blood pressure, and diabetes. Exercise can help control your blood sugar, lower your blood pressure, and, if you're obese, help you lose weight. Even a modest weight loss, such as twenty or thirty pounds, can lower blood pressure and improve the health of someone who is very heavy, say fifty to one hundred pounds overweight or even more.

But it is absolutely essential that you be evaluated before beginning any type of exercise program. This is because exercise affects your blood sugar level. Also, as a diabetic starting to exercise, you might miss the important sign of chest pain. So ask your doctor if an exercise stress test is in order.

These extra precautions may seem like a lot of trouble. But, when it comes to diabetes, the best defense is a good offense. Knowledge is power. Having the facts on your side gives you additional assurance that you'll lead a long, active life.

What You Can Do:
- Discuss with your doctor the best dietary plan to keep your blood sugar level under control. Consider consulting a nutritionist.
- See your doctor for regular checkups and make certain you notify your doctor of any changes you perceive in the way you feel.
- Be sure to monitor your blood sugar regularly. Home blood sugar monitoring has become accurate because of newer technology. For a good estimate of your overall control, a laboratory test called the hemoglobin A-1C has become widely available.

#10

INVOLVE YOUR FAMILY

When Ed suffered a heart attack, his thoughts centered on his son, Jon. A senior at an Ivy League college, Jon's final exams were coming up. Ed instructed his wife not to call Jon until after he was in recovery. Jon was furious at being left out during this time of crisis.

In her family, Ruth was known as the "stoic one." When she learned she had heart disease, she seemed to draw an emotional curtain around herself. "I'm always the one who holds the family together. I feel like I've let everyone down," she said.

The upshot? Both Ed and Ruth were in emotional pain, but they were not the only ones. Their families felt left out and helpless.

Heart disease does not only affect you, it affects your entire family. Coping with heart disease is a family affair.

According to Wayne Sotile, Ph.D., author of the book *Heart Illness and Intimacy*, the relationship between husband and wife is usually affected the most when heart disease strikes. Take Roberta, for example. "My husband developed a protective attitude about me which was driving me nuts. I just couldn't get him to realize that I was still the same person as I was before. He treated me like glass," she said.

Communication is crucial in family relationships all the time, but the need for it is greatest during or just after times of crisis. You may think only a heart attack or coronary bypass surgery warrants such classification, but being diagnosed with a potentially life-threatening illness like heart disease also certainly qualifies.

If you have young children, they may be frightened you will die. An honest discussion of what heart disease is, emphasizing the medical progress which has been made, can quell their fears. Thanks to modern developments in the treatment of heart disease, you can honestly answer that you expect to live a very long time.

If your children are grown, your diagnosis of heart disease may hit them surprisingly hard. Such a diagnosis may stir guilt feelings in them, or awaken a realization of your mortality (and theirs!). Since they're older, they may think it childish to express their concern. The stress they are under may manifest itself in other ways, such as chronic migraine headaches, constant worry, or irritability.

According to Dr. Sotile, the vast majority of the adult children living in the U.S. live within a two-hour drive of their parents. If they live close by, they may find themselves putting their own lives on hold. Sometimes, they'll make decisions not in their own best interests, or their parents' best interests, but on what they *think* their parents' best interests are, he notes. This also may occur if they live farther away. If they are driven by guilt, they may not make the best decisions.

Encourage your family members to express their fears and concerns. You may want to schedule a family conference with your doctor, so everyone can air their concerns and obtain firsthand information. Harriet, for example, was fearful when her husband, Bud, decided to return to his previous love of long-distance cycling after his heart attack. She relaxed when told by Larry's doctor that it was safe.

Family support is extremely important when making difficult lifestyle changes. Having a walking partner can make a big difference when you're trying to establish an exercise pattern. On the other hand, don't expect your partner to drop what they're doing because you want to take a walk. If you like to walk in the morning, but your spouse is not a morning person, compromise. Perhaps a late afternoon walk will suit you both. To encourage your spouse, give gifts of exercise clothing, club memberships, or sports equipment on special occasions. Find new activities you can do together; it can put zest back into your relationship.

If you do it as a family, the lifestyle changes you make can not only benefit you, but them as well. In the past, only men were considered vulnerable to heart disease, but now we know this is untrue. The lifestyle changes you make together will benefit your partner, too. If you have young children or teenagers, remember that although coronary artery disease is an adult ailment, researchers have found the beginning of telltale narrowing of the coronary arteries in individuals as young as fifteen! Use your heart disease experience to benefit your whole family. The heart-smart habits your youngsters develop now will stand them well in later life.

Encourage your kids (or your grandkids) to join you in exercising. Determine a regular exercise schedule and make it known you're sticking with it! This shows younger members of your family the importance of making time for exercise, not just fitting it in. Also, by exercising with your family, you show that it is a valuable and pleasurable habit.

Involving your family in your action plan can initially be difficult. Communicating sometimes can mean taking risks;

you don't always hear what you want. But achieving something as valuable as your family's wholehearted support can be well worth the risk.

What You Can Do:
- Ask your family members to read this book and help you initiate the "50 Things to Do." Read together other literature about heart disease. Sources are listed in the "Resources" section of this book.
- The American Heart Association sometimes sponsors activities which are perfect for the whole family, such as the annual walk-a-thon. Contact your local affiliate for more information.
- Facing a crisis such as heart disease can cause stress in the most loving of families. If your family has serious problems, health problems can be very damaging. If you, or your family members, seem unable to cope, consider talking to your doctor or a social worker about family counseling.

CHAPTER THREE

BE INFORMED

Knowing about heart disease is, of course, your doctor's job. But it is important that you keep up with medical developments as well, especially nowadays, when doctors are facing increasing limits in the amount of time they can spend with their patients. You need to know how to talk with your doctor in the most effective way possible to get the information you need. Also, you are likely to be faced with choices about your medical care. This is especially true in dealing with heart disease, when there is often more than one "correct" treatment. By keeping up with medical developments, you'll know the right questions to ask so you can make knowledgeable decisions about your heart's care.

The good news is that there has been a veritable explosion of medical information in the media. Nowadays, almost every newspaper has a health section. Health news is a staple on radio and television as well. But along with this information explosion has come a great deal of misinformation as well. The following sections are designed to help you learn to sort out the useful from the useless, and learn to discern the medical information which applies to you.

#11

KEEP UP WITH MEDICAL INFORMATION

If you've ever been part of a legal case, you know that no one is more expert about the details of your own case than you are. Your lawyer provides guidance, but has scores of other cases. Keep in mind the old adage, though, that "no one but a fool has himself for a lawyer."

This analogy applies to medicine as well. No one has more of an interest in keeping up with the latest medical developments in heart disease than you do. But just as you wouldn't represent yourself in a legal case, you wouldn't prescribe medicine for yourself either. The ultimate judge of what medical information is useful is your doctor.

But you should keep abreast of the latest medical advancements, and your doctor should welcome your interest. Even if what you learn doesn't apply in your own case, it can open the way to a useful discussion, and give you increased understanding about the active role you can play in your heart's care.

There are different ways to keep up with medical news.

Increasingly, a number of medical centers are publishing newsletters designed for the general public. These newsletters vary in style tremendously; some are technical in nature, while others are quite basic. They often contain articles about recent research in medical journals, but are written in more understandable language. A sampling of these newsletters are listed in the "Resources" section in the back of this book.

If you've got an analytical bent, you may want to sample some of the medical journals your doctor reads to keep up. There are several major medical journals, but two of the most popular, the *Journal of the American Medical Association* and the *New England Journal of Medicine,* are commonly found in most public or college libraries.

Usually, there's no need to directly delve into the medical literature. Nowadays, these studies are appearing on the evening news. Studies on heart disease in women, vitamin E, and the frequency of coronary bypass operations done on African Americans are all examples of research that appeared in journals but were published simultaneously in newspapers.

With so much information available in the media, it's necessary to separate the useless from the useful. Here are some guidelines:

- Be discriminating. New stories written by medical writers for such major publications as *The New York Times* are generally far more informative than those appearing in smaller newspapers or most tabloids.
- What kind of study is it? There are three types of medical studies: Experimental, epidemiologic, and clinical. Experimental studies are usually animal studies, which are often preliminary and need to be verified later using humans before researchers can determine if the findings are relevant at all. Epidemiologic studies make observations from a given group of participants over time, but do not involve

any intervention, or the taking of any action. An example is the Framingham Heart Study which identified cholesterol as a risk factor for heart disease. The participants were not forced to eat food high in cholesterol; the information was gleaned by analyzing their eating habits and whether they developed heart disease. Clinical studies are often used to back up observational studies before firm conclusions can be made or an intervention done. For example, one epidemiologic study, the Nurses' Health Study, found that estrogen lowered a woman's risk of heart disease. In a clinical study, some women would be given estrogen, and others not, to determine whether this was the factor that caused the benefit.

- Is this the first time these results have ever been reported? If so, it will take a while for studies to be done to confirm them. There is a big difference between the results of a single study or two and consensus statements based on many experiments reported by organizations like the American Heart Association.
- Do the findings make sense? If there is sound reasoning behind a finding, the chances are better it will hold up over time.
- Can the treatment be harmful? For example, studies have shown that drinking a moderate amount of alcohol is beneficial to a person's cholesterol level. Excessive drinking leads to a host of medical ailments and social ills, such as drunk driving and even suicide.

What You Can Do: Learn to use the many resources available for medical information. Visit your local library and learn how to access articles of interest in medical journals. If you are a computer enthusiast, investigate the many resources found in electronic on-line services such as The Internet, Compu-Serve, and America On Line.

#12

BE SKEPTICAL

Even highly intelligent people who have chronic conditions such as heart disease may be lured by marketers of unproven cures. But before you are tempted by the latest fad, wait. Sometimes these treatments will cost you plenty, but are essentially useless.

Today, there are many effective treatments and drugs on the market. It was not always that way. In the early days, medicine could offer little more than placebos. A placebo, defined as a substance without any active ingredients, may be a pill, sham surgery, or some other treatment. But, despite this, the patient often feels better. This is known as the placebo effect.

The power of the placebo effect is often discounted. But, as an August 1993 article in *The New York Times* noted, it may actually result in positive effects people experience in treatment trials as much as two-thirds of the time!

Proponents of quack cures use this placebo effect to their advantage. They offer testimonials from people who maintain they've been cured or that their condition has improved. Be skeptical. Evaluating a treatment for heart disease can be difficult. Symptoms such as chest pain tend to come and go. What appears to be the beneficial effect of a treatment might not necessarily be so. To know if a treatment really works, researchers subject it to scientific testing to eliminate the placebo effect.

As a heart patient, one so-called cure of which you should be skeptical is "chelation therapy." This involves the infusion of a chemical substance called ethylenediamine-tetraacetic acid (EDTA), which is used to remove heavy metals, such as lead, from the body and calcium from the blood. EDTA is most often used in the cases of heavy metal poisoning because of its ability to latch on to or bind these metals, creating a compound that can be excreted in the urine.

Besides binding heavy metals, EDTA also chelates (naturally seeks out and binds) to calcium, one of the components of the atherosclerotic plaque which causes the coronary arteries to narrow.

This once led to speculation that chelation therapy could be used as a kind of "magic bullet" to break up atherosclerotic plaque. However, there is no scientific evidence that chelation is effective. This therapy can be quite expensive. A course of treatments can cost thousands of dollars, according to the American Heart Association. In addition, experts warn that this type of therapy can also be dangerous. It's been linked to kidney failure, bone marrow depression, shock, low blood pressure, convulsions, heart rhythm irregularities, allergic reactions, and respiratory arrest.

Chelation therapy is not the only unproven cure touted for heart disease. In 1993, the Food and Drug Administration put pressure on companies that use unsubstantiated claims to tout their dietary supplements. As we note in this book, Vitamin E, as well as other vitamins known as antioxidants, are currently being subjected to rigorous scientific examination, and the early results are promising. But there are many other vitamin and nutritional supplements being marketed for which there is no such evidence.

Another therapy touted as a cure for heart disease, but lacking any scientific proof, is called "homeopathy." This is a type of treatment based on the idea that symptoms of a disease can be cured by administering minuscule amounts of substances that would in healthy people produce similar symptoms.

What You Can Do: In 1993, the National Institutes of Health established the Office of Alternative Medicine to scientifically test the claims made for these types of treatments. If you are interested in these methods, watch for those results. Until then, though, discuss treatments you are considering with your doctor.

CHAPTER FOUR

Know About Drugs, Vitamins, and Hormones

In the history of cardiology, the development of cardiovascular drugs may not seem as dramatic as the invention of procedures such as coronary bypass surgery or angioplasty, but it is indeed thanks to these drugs that many people with heart disease lead active lives. Another great area of interest to people with heart disease is vitamins. Research is now coming out that shows that some vitamins indeed may afford benefits when it comes to heart disease, although research is still ongoing. If you are a woman, you're probably aware of the issue of hormone replacement therapy, and you're wondering whether this treatment would help your heart. Read on for essential information on all these topics.

#13

TAKE YOUR MEDICINE

"Take your medicine." Sounds simple, but studies show many people do not take their cardiovascular medications, resulting in illness and even death. Some people simply refuse to take drugs, finding them "unnatural." This is ironic, as often these same people will down vitamins and nutritional supplements by the handful, not realizing that some can have adverse effects. Other people shy away from taking their pills because of the cost or unpleasant side effects.

It is essential you know about the type of drugs you are prescribed, what they do, and their potential side effects. Here's a brief look:

DRUGS FOR ANGINA PECTORIS (CHEST PAIN)

These drugs provide relief from the chest pain which sometimes accompanies heart disease:

Nitrates: Among the oldest heart medicines, nitrates provide temporary relief from chest pain by dilating your blood vessels. They are available in pill or capsule form, or as a skin patch.

Beta Blockers: These drugs block the effects of adrenaline, slow your heart rate, reduce the squeeze of your cardiac muscle, and lower your blood pressure.

Calcium-Channel Blockers: These drugs affect the squeeze of your heart and relax your blood vessels. They're also excellent at lowering high blood pressure and regulating irregular heart rhythms.

DIURETICS

Once prescribed alone, today diuretics are often used as a backup or in combination with other drugs to treat high blood pressure. They are also commonly used to help treat heart failure and fluid retention.

ACE INHIBITORS

Angiotensin Converting Enzyme inhibitors, commonly called ACE inhibitors, are effective in treating different types of heart problems, including treating congestive heart failure and high blood pressure.

CARDIAC STRENGTHENERS

These drugs are used to strengthen your heart muscle and improve its function. The major example is digoxin (Lanoxin), which can also be helpful in treating heart failure and controlling certain types of heart rhythm disturbances.

BLOOD THINNERS

The only commonly available blood thinner, wafarin (Coumadin and others), is a strong substance which interferes with your blood's normal coagulation. Wafarin is commonly used for people with mechanical heart valves or to prevent stroke in people who suffer from atrial fibrillation, a common type of heartbeat irregularity. Aspirin, although technically not a blood thinner, does block the formation of blood clots and is discussed in step 14 (page 61).

RHYTHM STABILIZERS

These correct an irregular heartbeat or slow your heart if it is beating too fast. Beta blockers, referred to earlier, are commonly used as rhythm-stabilizing drugs.

WHAT ABOUT GENERICS?

One of the objections many people have to taking cardiovascular drugs is their expense. So if you're watching your wallet (and who isn't?), you may wonder whether less expensive generic drugs are just as good for heart problems.

Many generic drugs provide the same, or nearly the same, therapeutic action as their brand-name counterparts. But, when it comes to heart drugs, you need to be very cautious, says Dr. Alan Bakst, of the Department of Hospital Pharmacy at the Cleveland Clinic. Some generic drugs may be acceptable, he points out. But some can cause problems, particularly those substances which must be maintained at certain critical levels in the blood to be effective. These include digoxin, quinidine, and wafarin. This does not necessarily mean you should rule out generic forms of these drugs. But your doctor should watch for any adverse effects.

In addition, generic drug formulas can vary slightly among manufacturers. So, if you are taking a generic drug, be sure to ask your pharmacist each time you get a refill whether the generic drug is made by the same company that made your previous prescription. If there has been a switch to another manufacturer, talk to your doctor so you can be on the lookout for any possible adverse effects. Also, if you are taking a brand-name drug, but would like to switch to a generic, discuss it first with your doctor.

TIPS FOR TAKING CARDIOVASCULAR DRUGS

- Take an inventory of all the drugs you have used in the last month, including over-the-counter and prescription drugs. When you see your doctor, *bring along the list*. You may find out you are taking too many medications or that some are inappropriate or redundant. The fewer drugs you need to take, the lower the possibility you'll develop side effects.
- Learn how much of the medication you should take, how often you should take it, and whether or not it should be taken with food. Be consistent with your schedule and dosages. Use pill organizers or dispensers if you need help in remembering to take your pills.
- Take exact doses as prescribed by your doctor. Never intentionally skip or add doses. Consult your doctor before you stop taking a cardiovascular medication. Keep your medicines in their original containers; don't mix them in the bottle with others.
- Take your medicine at the same time each day, at a time that is easy to remember, such as before meals, after work, or at bedtime.
- Do not take any over-the-counter (nonprescription) medications, such as aspirin, Alka-Seltzer, vitamins, and so on, without consulting your doctor or pharmacist. Many drugs can cause harmful interactions with others.
- Store your medicines at room temperature, away from moisture and out of direct sunlight. Don't store them on your bathroom sink or in your refrigerator. Some medications lose their strength after a few months; if a medication

is more than six months old, contact your doctor or pharmacist to determine if it should be discontinued or replaced.

- If you are going on a trip, plan ahead. Take twice as much medication with you as you would expect to need. Pack half of your drugs in your luggage; carry on your person a second supply which could last several days. This way, if your purse or carry-on is lost or stolen, you still have an adequate supply for your trip.

- It's very important to remember that your drugs are intended only for you, not your spouse, neighbor, or friend. Likewise, you should never take another person's medication.

- Many cardiovascular drugs are very powerful and may have side effects, such as fatigue, depression, fainting, and dizziness. If you experience such side effects, contact your doctor.

The point about cardiac drugs is the fact that they work. This can seduce you into thinking that your problem is cured. The reality is that this is the positive effect of the drug. Stop the drug, and the problem returns.

Many people resist being put on a drug indefinitely. If you're taking several medications, the scheduling can be complicated. But keep in mind that it is because of these drugs that the vast majority of people with heart disease live longer and lead the active lives they do.

What You Can Do:
- Discuss the drugs you take with your doctor. Once you verify you are taking the proper drugs, figure out an easy-to-remember schedule.
- Clean out your medicine chest. Throw out any drugs which have expired effectiveness dates. Flush them down the toilet, so children or animals can't come across them.

#14

An Aspirin-a-Day

For a drug that has been around for a century, aspirin was hailed anew as a wonder drug a few years ago. Studies showed its effectiveness in preventing heart attacks, particularly when taken by people who already have coronary artery disease. The hoopla stemmed from reports which showed that taking a daily aspirin could significantly reduce the risk of a heart attack.

How does aspirin work? A heart attack can occur when fatty plaque buildup in a blood vessel ruptures. When this happens, substances within the blood vessel lining can form a blood clot, blocking blood flow through the artery to the heart muscle, and causing a heart attack. Aspirin inhibits an important enzyme in that clotting process. So although taking an aspirin won't stop the progression of coronary heart disease, it can help stop blood clots from forming, lessening heart attack risk.

That said, the question remains: How much aspirin should you take?

A tiny amount of aspirin can inhibit this aspect of blood clotting in a test-tube. Your body, though, is not a test-tube. When aspirin is in your bloodstream, its effect varies, so the exact beneficial amount is difficult to establish. As little as 80 mg (a "baby" aspirin) may be effective. However, most cardiologists recommend taking one 325 mg pill (an adult aspirin) each day.

The least expensive type of generic aspirin that you can find will work. Many people find the enteric coated type preferable because they cause less stomach irritation. Remember, though, aspirin substitutes, such as acetaminophen (Tylenol) and ibuprofen (Advil) are not used for reducing platelet activity.

Although most people can safely take aspirin, not everyone can. If you have kidney problems, bleeding disorders such as hemophilia or low platelet count, or if you participate in hobbies or sports in which you may be injured, such as horseback riding and mountain climbing, consult a physician before starting to take aspirin on a regular basis to prevent heart attack. Of course, if you are allergic to aspirin, you should not take it.

In addition to preventing heart attacks, aspirin has also been shown to reduce the risk of stroke. If you've had a stroke, however, you should take aspirin only on your doctor's recommendation.

As important as aspirin may be in preventing heart attacks, you're only fooling yourself if you look upon it as a substitute for making other lifestyle changes, such as quitting smoking, losing excess weight, or exercising.

What You Can Do: Ask your doctor whether you should begin a daily aspirin regimen.

#15

CONSIDER TAKING VITAMIN E

Recently, vitamin E has been heralded as the latest weapon in the arsenal against heart disease. Although all of the evidence is not yet in, current research indicates that taking a daily vitamin E supplement may be useful.

Vitamin E is one of a group of vitamins called antioxidants. This means the vitamin helps counteract the effects of oxidation, the process that causes metal to rust, butter to turn rancid and, some researchers believe, that leads to the formation of fatty plaque buildup in the coronary arteries.

In May 1993, the *New England Journal of Medicine* reported studies involving both men and women which found that those who took daily vitamin E supplements had a significantly reduced risk of heart disease.

However, these studies are not considered conclusive. Although they involved a large number of participants, the results showed only an associative link between vitamin E and the reduced risk. This means the studies were not subjected to the rigorous double-blind technique that leads to conclusions beyond dispute.

Although concrete scientific proof is still lacking, these results show promise. Remember, though, that even though it is sold over-the-counter, vitamin E can be harmful to people with some medical conditions, or those taking some types of medications. For example, people with a rare deficiency of vitamin K can develop severe bleeding problems from large doses of vitamin E.

Many cardiologists, though, endorse the taking of vitamin E, and some take it themselves. What's the optimum dosage? Some preliminary studies indicate that a daily dose of 400 IU of vitamin E is safe and effective.

By the way, two other vitamins linked in this group of antioxidants, including beta carotene and vitamin C, were included in the studies published in the *New England Journal of Medicine*, but they were not found to be as effective as was vitamin E. More testing needs to be done.

If you don't want to take vitamin E, don't feel pressured to do so. But the studies indicate that this is something you should at least consider.

> *What You Can Do:* Ask your doctor if there is any reason why you should not take vitamin E. If not, consider taking a daily dose not to exceed 800 IU.
> • Watch the media for additional research findings about vitamin E. You can always reevaluate your decision to start (or stop) taking the vitamin based on the results of scientific research.

#16

FOR WOMEN ONLY: CONSIDER HORMONES

Since you have heart disease, you want to do everything you possibly can to prevent it from worsening, or leading to a heart attack. That's the major theme of this book. But whether or not, as a woman, you should take hormones is a sticky subject.

Major studies have shown that by taking estrogen, the female hormone, women can reduce their risk of heart disease. Although not all the evidence is in yet, many cardiologists find the studies very convincing. Yet taking hormones is not completely without risk. So there are some important things to keep in mind.

As women age and their estrogen decreases, they run a higher risk of dying from heart disease. It has not yet been determined exactly how estrogen works, but it appears to positively affect a woman's cholesterol profile, lessening the narrowing of the arteries that occurs with heart disease. Estrogen also helps prevent osteoporosis, the so-called "brittle-bone" disease which afflicts older women.

But the issue is not that clear-cut. For the past half-century, discussion has also centered on whether the pros of taking estrogen outweigh the cons. Estrogen replacement therapy fell into disrepute in the 1970s, when it was found to increase the risk of a woman's developing uterine or endometrial cancer. Since then, hormone replacement therapy has undergone a major change. Scientists discovered that combining estrogen with progesterone, the other hormone produced during a woman's menstrual cycle, greatly reduced this risk. This combination is now generally known as hormone replacement therapy, or HRT.

Most of the studies showing the positive effects of hormone on the heart had involved estrogen alone, but in 1994 results of a major study showed that the combination does help prevent heart disease. More research on this is underway. If you've undergone a hysterectomy, though, uterine cancer is no longer a threat, and you are a candidate for pure estrogen.

Another controversy surrounding both estrogen and HRT is whether they increase the risk of breast cancer and if so, by how much. The studies have been contradictory, but most studies indicate that long-term use of HRT does increase the risk of breast cancer. Most experts contend this increase is only slight, but some differ. Again, research in this area is also underway.

If you opt for HRT, follow the American Cancer Society's recommendation for mammograms and breast examinations. The address for the ACS is listed in the "Resources" section.

Until more research results are available, we will stop short of saying that it is essential that you undertake replacement hormone therapy. However, if you are a female with coronary heart disease, we believe you should seriously consider it, taking your individual risks and benefits into consideration.

What You Can Do:

- Discuss HRT with your doctor. To fully explore all your options, you may find that a second opinion is worthwhile.
- HRT is a subject that's too complicated to be fully dealt with here. There are some books which discuss the pros and cons of HRT. Some are listed in the "Resources" section at the back of this book.
- If you opt for replacement hormones, you can re-evaluate your decision as more information becomes available. Make sure you are on the lowest possible dosage considered sufficient to help protect your heart and bones.

CHAPTER FIVE

BE PREPARED

One of the most important things you can do for your heart is to be prepared in the event of a cardiac emergency. Since you have heart disease, you are at increased risk of suffering a heart attack. But, instead of living in fear, empower yourself. Learn the symptoms of a heart attack. Discuss with your doctor exactly what you should do in such an event. Map an emergency plan and make your family aware of it as well. The following sections will help you create your own strategy for dealing with an emergency.

#17

LEARN CPR
(AND ENCOURAGE
OTHERS TO DO
SO, TOO)

If you have heart disease, the people with whom you live and work could save your life. But they have to know how to perform CPR.

CPR, known otherwise as Cardiopulmonary Resuscitation or Basic Life Support (BLS) is a proven lifesaver. Just ask Louise, who was fifty-three when she suffered a heart attack while at work at her secretarial job at a car dealership. "The ambulance got lost on its way and no one arrived for twenty minutes. If my coworkers hadn't known CPR, they said I would've been a goner," Louise said.

If you are not medically trained, it is normal to doubt your capabilities in an emergency. Indeed, CPR was once considered only appropriate for medical personnel. But today, most lifeguards are required to learn CPR. Many communities now require it for high school graduation. People in all walks of life have enthusiastically learned the technique and are proud of their ability to use it if called upon in an emergency.

If you have severe heart disease, or are frail or disabled by another illness, ask your doctor if performing CPR would be dangerous for you. If it's not, consider learning it. Encourage your family and coworkers to learn it, too. They may someday help save your life, or you may do the same for them.

What You Can Do: Contact your local affiliate of the American Heart Association for a brochure which tells how to become trained in CPR. For added confidence, consider becoming BLS Certified. Contact your local community center or adult education program to learn when and where the next class is offered.

#18

Know What to Do When You Get Chest Pain

If you have heart disease, it is very likely that, because of it, you sometimes experience chest pain. Such chest pain can be unrelated to your heart, a normal part of your condition, or it can be an *important warning sign*.

The type of chest pain caused by coronary heart disease is called angina pectoris. This chest pain occurs when your heart muscle is trying to do its job, but is not receiving enough oxygen, usually because of a narrowing in a coronary artery. This type of angina is directly related to physical exertion. A second type, known as vasospastic angina, occurs during periods of rest, or may even awaken you from sleep. This type of angina results from a temporary spasm of the coronary artery, not from a permanent narrowing.

Often, chest pain occurs that is not related to the heart. One common cause of noncardiac chest pain is called esophageal dysfunction. Your esophagus, a muscular tube controlled by valves, carries liquid and chewed food from the back of your throat to your stomach. If the lower valve does not shut tightly enough, some of the acidic contents from your stomach can splash back, inflaming your esophagus and resulting in a sensation that feels like it comes from the heart.

Other noncardiac causes of chest pain include osteoarthritis of the neck. People with this type of "wear and tear" arthritis can develop bony spurs which dig into the nerves in their neck, and can cause pain which seems to come from the chest. Sometimes, spasms of the muscles of the chest wall, gas in the colon, shingles, and even stomach ulcers and gallbladder disease can feel like chest pain from the heart.

All of us experience chest pain at one time or another. On the one hand, if you have heart disease, or have suffered a heart attack, anxiety can magnify so-called normal aches and pains, making it impossible to sort out if your chest pain is from a cardiac cause or not. So, if you do experience chest pain, you should discuss this with your doctor. Your doctor will either give you the reassurance you need or decide on a further course of action if he or she suspects a problem.

Your doctor can also give you guidelines to help you plan what to do in the event your chest pain is due to a heart problem. Don't procrastinate. Nobody wants to face the possibility that something may be amiss. For men, it may be a "macho" thing. Women, on the other hand, sometimes tend to delay getting help because they are afraid of the potential impact of a heart emergency on their families.

Chest pain may be your heart's warning you that something is wrong. Don't panic, but don't ignore it, either.

What You Can Do: Pay attention to your chest pain. Evaluate it so you know when it occurs and whether it is more frequent or severe. Discuss with your doctor whether or not you should take nitroglycerin when you experience chest pain. If your physician has given you a prescription for rapidly acting nitroglycerin, be absolutely sure you know when and how to take it and what to do if it doesn't work. If the pain is new, a change in your usual pattern, or the pain doesn't respond to what your physician has prescribed, follow the emergency plan you've discussed with your doctor in advance. Read on for how to create an emergency plan.

#19

MAP AN
EMERGENCY PLAN

If you suspect you are experiencing a heart attack, you need to take fast action. By acting quickly, you may be able to take advantage of new treatments that could not only save your life, but spare your heart damage. With heart disease you are at increased risk of suffering a heart attack, so it is crucial to have an "emergency plan" mapped out and ready for use.

There are some important things you can do to prepare for an emergency. First, you should discuss with your doctor what specific steps he or she would want you to take. This chapter can serve as an important springboard to such a talk. Discuss the steps outlined in this chapter, and see if your doctor wants you to modify any.

Second, you should carry a copy of your EKG (also known as an ECG) printout with you at all times. This is an electronic graphing of your heartbeat. If you have heart disease, if you've undergone heart surgery, or if you ever suffered a heart attack, these tracings may be normal for you, but appear markedly abnormal to someone who does not know your medical history. Ask your doctor for a copy of your most recent EKG. Having a copy of your EKG can be helpful should you ever be taken to the hospital. This way, it can be quickly ascertained whether your EKG results are indeed in the normal range for you, or whether you may be suffering a cardiac emergency. Mapping out such an emergency plan could very well save your life.

In the old days, if you were suffering a heart attack, it was important to get to the hospital quickly, so doctors could stabilize your condition and possibly save your life by treating complications of the attack. Yet there was nothing to do except let the heart attack run its course, resulting in whatever damage to your heart muscle that occurred. Nowadays, it is possible to stop a heart attack in its tracks, and minimize the heart muscle damage. But treatment is available only if you get help quickly.

The development of a class of drugs known as thrombolytics has caused this momentous change in treatment. These are known also as "clot busters." A heart attack usually occurs when a blood clot forms within a coronary artery and cuts off the supply of oxygen-filled blood to the heart. Clot-busters are powerful drugs which act to dissolve the clot, enabling the flow to resume. But they must be administered quickly.

There are different types of clot dissolvers. Tissue plasminogen activator, or tPA, is one type; another is streptokinase. What is important to remember is that if you've been given streptokinase before, you should be given tPA, because using streptokinase a second time could result in a severe allergic reaction. If you're African American, you should know that while both drugs work for you, research shows tPA to be more effective.

If a cardiac emergency arises, you should:

- Never attempt to drive yourself to the hospital. In general, studies have found that calling 911 is the quickest method to get help. This may differ in some communities, so discuss this with your physician.
- If you call 911, or a similar emergency number, tell the dispatcher that you think you're having a heart attack. Give the dispatcher your exact street location. Make certain your house is posted with a clearly visible number, and specify the floor, room or apartment number. Turn on the outside lights if it's dark out.
- Contact your cardiologist immediately. The cardiologist's number should be kept by every telephone in the house. Discuss with your cardiologist beforehand whether he or she may be best contacted at the office or at the clinic or hospital.
- If you arrive at the hospital's emergency room on your own, clearly state that you may be suffering a heart attack. This is especially important for women, since studies have shown that doctors sometimes overlook heart disease in women. If it turns out you are not having a heart attack, so much the better. But, since, as a woman with heart disease, you are at risk, you do not want to deprive yourself of potentially life-saving treatment.
- As a heart patient, you are also at increased risk for stroke as well. As with heart attacks, it used to be thought that nothing much could be done immediately for a stroke. But treatment with clot dissolvers is also being found effective for strokes. If you think you may be having a stroke, follow the same advice to get help quickly.

What You Can Do: Know the symptoms of a heart attack. You may be having a heart attack if:
- Chest pain comes on suddenly over a minute or two and builds in intensity.
- The pain occurs near the center of your chest.

- The pain lasts at least twenty minutes and is not relieved by rest or by changing position.
- The pain ranges from mild to severe, and usually feels like tightness or heaviness.
- The pain radiates up into your jaw, your back, or down your left arm.
- You experience nausea, shortness of breath, or a sense of "impending doom."
- It is important to remember that these are the common symptoms of a heart attack in both men and women. Studies have shown, however, that women often experience more subtle symptoms such as indigestionlike discomfort or difficulty breathing.

You may be having a stroke if you experience:

- Sudden weakness or numbness of the face, arm, or leg on one side of the body.
- Sudden difficulty speaking or understanding others.
- Dimness or impaired vision in one eye.
- Loss or near loss of consciousness.
- Confusion.
- Unexplained dizziness or sudden falls, especially along with any of the above symptoms.

A person who is faced with an impending stroke may suffer a TIA, a transient ischemic attack, or mini-stroke. The symptoms are the same as a stroke, but their duration is brief, usually from several minutes to a half-hour. If you experience what may be a TIA, also get help immediately.

#20

CHOOSE THE RIGHT HOSPITAL

In an emergency, you do not have the luxury of choosing a hospital; you must go to the closest available. But many times heart procedures are elective, which means they are not done on an emergency basis. Since a main theme of this book is "be prepared," you should know how to choose the right hospital in the event you need one.

If you require heart surgery, or an angioplasty-type procedure, you may select your doctor first. In doing so, you will be choosing the hospital where that physician is permitted to practice. On the other hand, you may have a particular hospital in mind; then you will be choosing among the doctors who practice there. Either way is fine, as long as you are making the best decision for *you*. Bear in mind that your future well-being may very well depend on your decision. You may be tempted to choose a hospital which is close by to minimize the inconvenience to your family. This is fine, but make sure you'll be getting the best medical care there as well.

Comparing hospitals isn't easy. As health care gets more competitive, hospitals are using more advertising and making more grandiose claims. Check them out carefully. Be wary of hospitals that tout themselves as "heart centers" but really have limited cardiac offerings. There should be at least two surgical teams available, for example, in the event a member of the team becomes ill or goes on vacation. Also, if you need to undergo cardiac catheterization, be careful about catheterization laboratories which claim to perform "low risk" procedures. In the event of an emergency, angioplasty or surgery may become necessary, and these labs often lack the facilities to perform them.

Experts agree that there is a *minimum* number of procedures that should be performed in a hospital in order for them to be competently performed. They are:

• Cardiac catheterization (also known as coronary angiography)—300 per year.
• Balloon angioplasty—200 per year.
• Coronary bypass surgery—150 per year.

Bear in mind that many hospitals tout "laser" angioplasty, giving the impression that this high-tech treatment is available for coronary artery disease when it really isn't. Coronary "laser" angioplasty is still an experimental technique, performed in only a few places in the country.

If you are at higher-than-average risk for cardiac procedures, then you might want to consider a regional or even a national heart health center. How do you know if you fit this description? Discuss it with your doctor. Factors that increase risk include:

• Whether your heart has been previously damaged by a heart attack or other cause.

- You have multiple heart problems, such as both heart disease and a faulty heart valve.
- You underwent open-heart surgery before (particularly if you did not do well).
- You have other potentially complicating medical problems such as diabetes and/or high blood pressure.
- You're over sixty-five years of age. Open-heart surgery is now being done successfully in people in their seventies or even eighties, but the risk is higher.
- You're a woman. Cardiac procedures are effective and may be lifesaving for a woman, but being female also may increase your risk of complications.

To find directories of institutions of excellence, check the "Resources" section. You can call these institutions directly for information. They usually have toll-free 800 numbers. Contrary to what many people think, you can often refer yourself. If you live far away, you can sometimes send your medical records or test results for evaluation. Check your health insurance, though, to make sure you'll be covered.

What You Can Do: Visit the hospitals in your area. Learn their areas of expertise. Knowing you've selected your ideal hospital, should you ever need it, will give you peace of mind.

CHAPTER SIX

KNOW WHAT
TO EAT

The kind of food you eat can make a difference in your fight against heart disease. That you must stick to a low-fat diet probably does not come as a surprise, but it probably does not come as welcome news either. Some people don't care about what they eat and can easily adapt to a strict diet. Many of us, though, consider good food to be one of life's pleasures, and we fear that having heart disease will sentence us to a life of stiff food restrictions. This really isn't the case at all. What you need to know is how to create a delicious eating plan that will stay within the low-fat guidelines and will help you in your fight against heart disease. Impossible, you say? Read on.

#21

LEARN ABOUT CHOLESTEROL

For the past several years, there's been a national debate over whether all Americans should be concerned about their level of cholesterol. Once you've been diagnosed with heart disease, though, the debate's over. Most people with heart disease have some type of cholesterol problem. So if your cholesterol level is too high, you need to lower it.

First, though, you should know exactly what cholesterol is, and how too high levels contribute to heart disease. The more understanding you have, the easier it is to take action.

A pearly, fatlike substance, cholesterol is an essential component of your body. It is found in the membranes of your cells, used in the formation of the bile acids that digest your food, and even contributes to your sex hormones. You need cholesterol in your blood to live. However, too much cholesterol is dangerous.

When we first learned about the importance of cholesterol levels, knowing your total cholesterol "number" was stressed. But today we know it's a little more complicated than that. What you need to know is the levels of the components that make up that total cholesterol figure. This is called your cholesterol profile.

The components which make up the cholesterol total include:

- High density lipoprotein, also called HDL-cholesterol
- Low density lipoprotein, also called LDL-cholesterol
- Triglycerides

LDL-cholesterol is the so-called "bad" cholesterol. This substance contributes to the development of heart disease by depositing itself in the arterial wall, forming the fatty streaks that can progress to the narrowing of the arteries. On the other hand, HDL-cholesterol, the so-called "good" cholesterol, reduces the accumulation of cholesterol by transferring it away from the artery and blocking the initial steps in plaque formation. In a sense, it's like having a drain cleaner cleansing your arteries. Triglycerides are fatty compounds found in combination with LDL-cholesterol, and are increasingly implicated in contributing to coronary artery disease.

If your blood cholesterol level is undesirable, your doctor will most likely recommend you try changing it through diet and exercise. If it is severely high or cannot be controlled this way, your doctor will probably prescribe one of the cholesterol-lowering drugs on the market.

Does a low-fat diet really reduce cholesterol?

The low-fat, low-cholesterol diet is a bedrock of modern heart-health. You can't go through a day without hearing on the television or radio something about how to eat a low-fat diet. Yet this diet is the bane of both doctors and those afflicted with cholesterol problems. After the stern, requisite lecture from your doctor, you may find that after eight to twelve weeks of really serious trying, your LDL-cholesterol has hardly budged, and the HDL-cholesterol, which is often lower than desirable to start with, actually goes down (the wrong direction!). If this is the case, why bother with the diet at all?

Research shows that if you have a severe cholesterol problem, a low-fat diet and a cholesterol-lowering drug in combination is the most effective way to lower your cholesterol; for many people, it's better than either alone. Cholesterol-lowering drugs, such as lovastatin, do most of their work inside the cells of the liver, where the drug interacts with your body's cholesterol. This process, experts believe, is activated by low-fat intake and depressed by diets high in fat. So, if you eat a high-fat diet, the drug is far less effective.

What's the impact of lowering your cholesterol? Since you have heart disease, the stakes are high. According to studies, if you have a total cholesterol level of 300 and reduce it to just 270 (a 10 percent reduction), you've reduced your risk of a heart attack by 20 percent!

You may wonder if you should take advantage of the cholesterol tests done in shopping malls and other public places. Don't bother. These "fingerstick" tests most often look at the total cholesterol level only and studies show the results can vary widely with the technique used.

Some people play a cat-and-mouse game with their cholesterol number; they are careful about what they eat before they go to the doctor and cheat afterward. This doesn't work, because it really takes several weeks for LDL and HDL levels to change. If you have a cholesterol problem, use the tips in this book to adopt long-range eating strategies you can live with.

What You Can Do: Find out from your doctor what your current cholesterol profile is and compare it to the level your doctor recommends. Do this each time your cholesterol profile is taken and use it to gauge your success on the program your doctor has designed for you.

Guidelines for Cholesterol Levels

Level	Classification
Total Cholesterol (mg/dL)	
200 or less	Desirable
200–239	Borderline-to-high
240 or more	Too high
LDL-Cholesterol (mg/dL)	
130 or less	Desirable*
130–159	Borderline-to-high
160 or more	Too high
HDL-Cholesterol (mg/dL)	
35 or more	Desirable

Adapted from the Second Report of the National Cholesterol Education Program Expert Panel on Detection, Evaluation, and Treatment of High Blood Cholesterol in Adults, *Journal of the American Medical Association*, vol. 269, No. 23, 1993.

*If you have coronary heart disease, optimal LDL-cholesterol would be 100 mg/dL or less.

Source: *Heartline*

#22

Eat to Lower Cholesterol

As we noted in the preceding section, some cholesterol exists normally in your body. But your body also gets cholesterol from the foods you eat. Only foods of animal origin—for example, meat, milk, and egg yolks, have cholesterol. Organ meats (liver, kidney, sweetbread, and brain) have the highest amounts of cholesterol.

There are two types of dietary fat: saturated and unsaturated. All foods that contain fat have a mixture of these two types.

Saturated fat raises blood cholesterol more than anything else you can eat. Animal fats that are solid at room temperature contain high amounts of saturated fats. Some vegetable oils also can be saturated (or hardened) by hydrogenation. Examples of saturated fats (the most important to stay away from) include butter, lard, meat fat, shortening, and hydrogenated oils such as palm and coconut oil, palm kernel oil, and cocoa butter.

Now what about margarine? Many people were con-

fused when studies came out which focused on the un-
healthful effects of margarine. Most of us turned to margarine years ago, when butter was condemned as unhealthy.
Well, the problem with margarine is that it is "hydrogenated," or hardened. This process produces trans fatty acids,
which some studies have also linked to an increased risk of
heart disease. If you're practicing heart-smart eating, the
American Heart Association maintains margarine is still better than butter and soft margarines are better than hard stick
forms. Choose a margarine with no more than two grams of
saturated fat per tablespoon. On the other hand, eating unsaturated fats, in moderation, in place of saturated fats can
lower your blood fat levels. Oils from plant products that are
liquid at room temperatures contain unsaturated fats. These
include safflower, sunflower, soybean, sesame, cottonseed
and corn oils. Fats high in monosaturated fats include canola
oil and peanut oils.

   Here are suggestions on how to lower the amount of
cholesterol you're eating from Andrea Vegh Dunn, a registered, licensed dietitian with the Cleveland Clinic Foundation's Nutrition Services Department.

• Choose low-fat dairy products, like skim or 1 percent milk,
  nonfat or low-fat yogurts and cheeses containing three
  grams of fat or less per ounce, if you intend to eat a one-
  ounce serving.
• Be a label reader. Limit those products that contain oil and
  fat as a first ingredient. Avoid foods that don't specify the
  type of vegetable oil used. These oils could be coconut,
  palm kernel or palm oil, which are more saturated.
• When buying meat, choose from poultry, fish, and lean
  meats such as chuck or tenderloin. Choose "select" and
  "choice" grades of meat instead of the "prime" cuts which
  have fat marbled into them. Remember, even poultry, fish,

and lean meats contain some fat and cholesterol, so eat them moderately.

What You Can Do: Educate yourself. Read labels and become a smart consumer.

To lower blood cholesterol levels:
- Limit cholesterol to 300 mg or less a day.
- Eat less fat, especially saturated fat.
- Replace saturated fats with unsaturated fats.
- Eat more complex carbohydrates and fiber.
- Achieve and maintain a good body weight.

Source: *Heartline*

#23

Lose Those Extra Pounds

It's no wonder that d-i-e-t is a four-letter word. Nobody likes to do it. And why should you? After all, if you're considering earthly pleasures, good food is definitely on the list.

But, if you're overweight, that extra bulk you are carrying around not only hampers your appearance, it's dangerous for your heart. So here's the essential news about losing weight. Keep in mind it is information that both authors of this book have used to trim down. And we are both food lovers!

First, eliminate the word "diet" from your vocabulary. It really *is* a four-letter word! And if you are like many women (and some men), simply contemplating a diet can kick in old compulsive eating habits that will send you scurrying to the refrigerator. Also, a diet implies that this is a temporary regimen. We prefer to think in terms of "eating plans" or "eating strategies." Since studies show that the vast majority of diet plans do not work, we suggest you create an eating plan for yourself by making subtle adjustments in the types of food you normally eat.

For example, if you customarily enjoy a muffin for breakfast, you won't stick with a diet that offers cold cereal instead for long. Substitute a low-fat muffin. This way, you can eat low-fat, and have your muffin, too! You can create a realistic eating plan so close to your normal habits that, unlike a diet, you have nothing "to go off of."

Consider giving the bathroom scale the old heave-ho. For many women especially, jumping on the scale can be so anxiety provoking it sends them to the refrigerator. Concentrate on your health, instead of your weight. Also, if you're exercising, you're building muscle. Muscle weighs more than fat, so your weight reading may be deceptive.

Be realistic. We are not advocating that you slim down to some unrealistic weight. Women especially tend to be overly critical of themselves and, even at their ideal weight, see themselves as too fat. Set realistic goals for yourself.

Take your time. It takes a while for your body to adjust to these new ways of eating, and for them to become a habit.

Count fat grams, not calories. We were all taught, years ago, that "a calorie is a calorie is a calorie," but that is not really the case. Fat really is more fattening, as you'll learn in our section entitled "Trim the Fat."

Watch your portion size. If you're trying to lose weight, the size of your servings count. Use a set of measuring cups, measuring spoons, or a small scale to get an idea of the size of the portions you are eating. Check to make sure no "portion inflation" has crept in.

Exercise is essential. When it comes to losing weight, many experts now believe that the exercising you do is even more important than what you do—or don't—eat. Exercise is also an excellent way to minimize stress, and studies show that particularly women, when they are under stress, tend to overeat.

Some people prefer to join a program to lose weight instead of doing it by themselves. If you're looking for support in changing your eating habits, you may find it at a cardiac rehabilitation program. If you decide to join a weight reduction program, here are some tips from a group of experts convened in 1992 by the National Institutes of Health:

- Don't be distracted by anecdotal "success" stories or advertising claims. Find out the percentage of beginning participants who complete the program, how much weight they lost, and how much weight loss they maintained one, three, or even five years later. If they can't supply this data, that's an especially bad sign. Also, find out the percentage of participants who experienced adverse health or psychological effects.
- What is the relative mix of diet, exercise, and behavior-modification methods used?
- What kind of counseling is used? Studies have found that counseling in "closed" groups (where membership generally doesn't change) is more effective than in groups where members come and go. Also, what are the qualifications of the program's leaders?
- A lot of people who lose weight are prone to regain it. Is there training done to promote maintenance of weight loss?
- How flexible is the food plan and is it suitable to your lifestyle and preferences?

Remember, as a heart patient, you must maintain good nutrition. This goal cannot be sacrificed for quick weight loss.

To be successful, studies have shown that losing weight slowly is the key. Don't plan on losing more than one or two pounds a week. Starving yourself on a low-calorie diet will leave you feeling deprived and increase the temptation to binge. You'll also lose muscle instead of fat.

We live in a quick-fix society. Ignore the barrage of television ads which tout fad and liquid diets. Hang in there! Your weight will come off and, most importantly, stay off.

What You Can Do: If you believe you are a compulsive eater, take a look at some of the books on the market about eating disorders and compulsive eating. Also, commit the steps outlined in this chapter to memory. They are:

- Eliminate the word "diet" from your vocabulary.
- You're not "dieting" to "lose weight," you are adopting new eating strategies for healthy living!
- Be realistic.
- Take your time.
- Exercise. (Read on for how to exercise safely.)

24

Trim the Fat

"I never get to eat anything good anymore. 'They' won't let me." "Everything that tastes good is bad for you!" "It's no use. No matter what I like, eventually 'they' will tell me it's bad for me."

These are often-heard complaints from people with heart disease. Sometimes, their gripe isn't with the "experts," but with their spouse, who is apt to glare at them if so much as the thought of a french fry crosses their mind.

Take back control of your eating. Being resentful isn't going to help. Besides, most likely, your ideas about "heart-healthy" eating were shaped years ago. Nowadays, more people are health conscious when it comes to mealtime. Okay, maybe not all of your favorite foods are on the "heart-healthy" list. But you can still enjoy a wide variety of foods. The key to this personal transformation lies in knowing how to "trim the fat."

Depending on which statistics you follow, Americans

derive from 37 percent to 50 percent of their daily calories from fat. The American Heart Association now recommends that people with heart disease allow no more than 30 percent of their daily calories to come from fat. Some experts claim that this total should be even lower, possibly down to 10 percent. Such drastic dietary changes are difficult for most people to maintain. Until these studies are done, your aim should be to eat the least amount of calories from fat as possible, while enjoying a healthy eating plan you can live with.

You may have learned that "a calorie is a calorie is a calorie." Technically, that's true. But the great thing about cutting out fat is you can actually feel like you're eating more, even though you are eating fewer calories. One gram of fat contains nine calories, but carbohydrates and protein contain only four calories each. So, every time you choose protein or carbohydrates instead of fat, you are saving five calories per gram consumed. Alcohol, by the way, has seven calories per gram. So, if you decide to have a drink, keep in mind you're consuming extra calories.

If you're just starting to keep track of your fat grams, you should evaluate how many fat grams you are eating, to make sure you are staying within that 25 to 30 percent calories from fat or lower. Opposite is a chart from *Heartline*, the newsletter published by the Coronary Club from the Cleveland Clinic Foundation, so you can readily recognize how to evaluate fat consumption.

DESIRABLE WEIGHTS/CALORIE LEVELS
FOR ADULTS AGES 55–74*

WOMEN

Height	Weight** (pounds)	Calories Needed Per Day***	Grams of Fat Equal to 30% of Calories
4'11"	136	1545	52
5'1"	141	1600	53
5'3"	143	1625	54
5'5"	147	1670	56
5'7"	158	1795	60
5'10"	161	1830	61

MEN

Height	Weight** (pounds)	Calories Needed Per Day***	Grams of Fat Equal to 30% of Calories
5'4"	156	1775	59
5'6"	163	1850	62
5'8"	172	1950	65
5'10"	176	2000	67
6'	178	2025	68
6'2"	209	2375	79

*Extrapolated from published data.
For medium frame without clothes or shoes:
**Add 10% for large frame, subtract 10% for small frame.
***May vary by ±400 calories/day depending on activity.

Source: *Heartline*

Bear in mind that, although you're counting fat grams, calories are not completely irrelevant. Many of the "no-fat" desserts, such as cakes and brownies, may not contain fat, but they do contain calories. If you indulge in them regularly, instead of just as an occasional treat, you may gain, not lose, weight.

Here are some easy ways to cut the fat in your eating:

- Cut down on your meat intake. This includes not just red meat, but chicken and fish as well. Most studies show Americans eat far too much meat. For example, reducing your meat consumption by two ounces daily will reduce your daily calories by 110. We don't advocate eliminating meat completely, but many people get along without any meat at all as long as they get enough protein from other sources, such as beans and lentils. Although cutting down on meat is one of the easiest ways to cut down on fat, many people find a vegetarian diet too restrictive. If you do, limit but don't necessarily eliminate meat. For example, instead of using beef or chicken as the main course, and vegetables or pasta as the side dish, switch. A three-ounce portion of fish, for example, accompanied by a large serving of vegetables and a hefty salad can be very filling indeed.
- Plan ahead. It's very difficult to eat healthy if it's noon, you're starved, and the only store in the area is a convenience store with a food section the size of a telephone booth. If you're on the road, know ahead of time which restaurant offers a full menu with heart-healthy alternatives, instead of just fried food. If you're home, make sure your cupboards and freezer are stocked with reduced-fat foods you enjoy.
- Become a culinary adventurer. The traditional American "meat-and-mashed potatoes with gravy" cuisine is not heart healthy. Leave your preconceived food notions at the door and delve into cookbooks from other countries. There

are wonderful meat-free dishes which can be made from lentils and different kinds of beans found in Indian, Mexican, Middle-Eastern, and Southwestern cookbooks, for example. Learn to cut down on the fat and oil in these recipes. Remember, though, just because it's ethnic doesn't mean it's low-fat. Take Chinese food, for example. Egg rolls, fried rice, and spare ribs are laden with fat. But eating stir-fried dishes as they were intended, with plenty of steamed (not fried) rice, can be quite low-fat.

• If you are cooking ground beef, follow these tips. Have the butcher grind "extra lean" (15 percent fat); sauté, and then rinse the browned beef with warm water. This reduces the fat by another 5 to 7 percent.

• Wild game such as deer (venison), elk, and moose are red meats that are very low in fat. Red meats such as buffalo, range-fed ("unfinished") beef, and a buffalo/beef cross called "beefalo" are becoming increasingly available. These may have fat contents between 5 and 10 percent.

• Get the farm-fresh habit. If you live on the West Coast, you're fortunate to be able to get farm-fresh fruits and vegetables year-round. In other parts of the country, the months where "native" foods are available are times to be savored. Visit your local farms in season, and reap the harvest. The finest chefs in the land agree: There is nothing so delicious as a plump, juicy ripe native tomato dusted with chopped fresh basil leaves. Or bite into a farm-fresh ear of corn; there's no need to slather it in butter. If you're city bound, don't despair. Urban "farm markets" are a growing trend.

• Take advantage of fat-free and reduced-fat foods. Years ago, the pickings over in the "diet foods" category were pretty dismal. But food marketers have caught on that "fat free" means dollars, and now, there are absolutely delicious low-fat, and even no-fat, frozen yogurt, puddings, and even cakes available. Some of these are so good they will even fool the most dedicated gourmet. But you need to be a careful label-reader. And remember, "low-fat" and "no-fat" do not necessarily mean "no calories." Don't increase your intake because of the lower fat content.

What You Can Do:
- Learn to calculate the fat in your food by checking out the label, the recipe, or a fat-counter guidebook.
- Keep track of your food selection over a period of days. It's *over time* that your food choices should be within the 30-percent-from-fat guideline, not item by item.

#25

Become Supermarket Savvy

Over the past few years, eating heart-smart became a fad. In fact, the food industry began going after the market of health-conscious Americans so aggressively that soon nearly every food product was emblazoned with words like "low-fat" and "lite." It became so confusing that Congress stepped in, ordering food processors to adopt standardized labels. These are the black-and-white labels entitled "Nutrition Facts." By now, the vast majority of processed foods on your supermarket's shelves should be carrying this welcome label.

What does this label mean to you?

First of all, the label was designed to deter confusing claims that have resulted in many packaged and processed foods being adorned with misleading "fat-free" labeling. It provides you with a wealth of information so you can make informed choices about the type of foods you eat, and helps you compare food items.

The new labels list the serving size, amount of calories,

total fat, total carbohydrates, dietary fiber, protein, saturated fat, cholesterol, sodium, and a selection of vitamins and minerals, vitamin A, vitamin C, calcium and iron. The label also shows how the food fits into a 2,000- and a 2,500-calorie diet. If you're a woman, this calorie count may be too high. But it does give you some perspective.

Take a careful look at the label. Serving size is obviously very important. Will you be satisfied with a small one-ounce square of low-fat cake, for example, or would three cups of microwaved popcorn with the same amount of fat better suit you? These are the types of decisions reading labels can help you make.

The total amount of calories derived from fat is the most important feature on the label. Aim for small numbers here. Under the category "total fat," you should find no more than 20 percent of the calories derived from fat. The label also lists "saturated fat." This is the most undesirable fat because of the role it plays in raising blood cholesterol. Choose foods which have no, or very little saturated fat. This goes also for the next listing, "cholesterol," which also leads to heart disease. The American Heart Association recommends you eat less than 300 mg of cholesterol per day.

The label also lists sodium content, a boon for those people who need to monitor salt intake because of high blood pressure. The heart association recommends healthy adults consume no more than 3,000 mg or less each day. If you are salt sensitive, aim for a lower amount.

The "Nutrition Facts" label does not list "trans fatty acids," a substance found in margarine as well as sometimes in other foods such as cakes, cookies, and crackers—even if they're labeled "low fat." Trans fatty acids have been implicated in causing heart disease. If the amount of unsaturated fat and saturated fat doesn't add up to the "total fat" figure, chalk the missing amount up to the presence of trans fatty acids. Also, check the ingredients list; if it includes partially hydrogenated oils or fats, the product contains trans fatty acids.

Once you get the hang of it, scanning a package will take no more than a few seconds. It will provide you with valuable information, even for choosing the type of chocolate chip cookie that might actually be "good" for you!

What You Can Do: Compare the Nutrition Facts label on different brands of the types of food you normally buy. Take along a pencil and paper; you may find that you'll be able to substitute lower-fat brands without making any significant changes in your eating preferences at all.

#26

Practice "Fat Banking"

We don't know about you, but we find it impossible to proclaim that we will *never* eat anything sinful again. Some people can do this; if you're one of them, great. But the minute we say, "I'm never going to eat another french fry" or "No more chocolate bars for as long as I live," that signifies the beginning of trouble. The world suddenly looks like a chocolate bar, or smells like a giant french fry.

The way to solve this problem is to learn "fat banking." This is an unbeatable technique for being able to chow down some extra fat grams, whether you're on a cruise, going to a special event like a wedding, or simply are beset by an impossible craving.

The principle of fat banking is simple. It's also essential, because it will make your eating plan adaptable to the temptations we face in real life.

Picture your calorie and fat allotments as the "balances" in your checking account. You can "draw" on these amounts just as you would a real bank account. So, say you go to that wedding and are faced with what you estimate is a hunk of sirloin or a wedge of buttercream-frosted wedding cake, each "weighing" in at about 15 fat grams. Using the checkbook analogy, that's like going into a store and falling in love with an expensive dress or set of golf clubs. You can deal with this dilemma in one of two ways. If you know ahead of time that you're going to want to spend these fat grams, you could have decreased your fat gram count by being extra careful the week before. That way, you can enjoy the extra fat grams now, just as if you had spent a month budgeting and bought that dress or golf clubs.

There is also another way to handle such a dilemma. Say you had planned to go to the wedding, but you believed you were going to have enough willpower to pass up the goodies. But now, it's just too tempting. Go ahead! You may be "overdrawing" on your calorie balance today, but it's only a temporary measure. Be extra careful for the next days. Voilà! You've got a balanced metabolic checkbook again!

Remember, you don't have to eat a total diet of low-fat foods. If occasionally you want to eat a meal which contains a high-fat "no-no," like a chunk of steak, there are some steps you can take to put your mind at ease.

First, limit the amount of the high-fat food you eat; with steak, for example, it should be about four ounces (about the size of a deck of cards). Second, balance the meal with low-fat choices. For example, if you want a small steak for dinner, enjoy it, but eat your baked potato sans butter, fill up on veggies, and choose fresh fruit for dessert. Third, keep track of your selection; pick low-fat choices for the next couple of days to balance the higher fat food you ate. That's guilt-free eating! You can have your steak and be virtuous too!

What You Can Do: Practice fat banking. Keep track of your choices carefully. Before you know it, it will become second nature.

27

LEARN TO COOK
"SPA CUISINE"

If you love to cook, you may feel the pleasures of the kitchen are now out of bounds. Not so! You'll find the cookbook section of your local bookstore lined with books featuring heart healthy foods that are geared to everyone from the most rudimentary to the gourmet chef. We're not talking about recipes that begin, "take two cups of cream and a stick of butter." But we'll make you a promise: Once you get accustomed to eating healthier, those recipes will not appeal to you as much anymore.

Bear in mind, according to food historians, heavy sauces were devised in the Middle Ages to disguise spoilage. Now that's not very appetizing, is it? Cooking light can be terrific. The in-name for this type of chic cooking is "spa cuisine." Here are some tips from Terry Frank Montlick, owner of the former Wood Creek Cooking School in Bethlehem, Connecticut.

• Rather than trying to leave out salt, sugar, and fat from existing recipes, switch to recipes which naturally use less of these ingredients.

- Sauté or grill foods, rather than fry, to use less fat or oil. If sautéeing, use a nonstick frying pan with a small amount of vegetable oil, such as olive oil.
- Learn the delights of outdoor grilling. Use an outdoor grill instead of an oven broiler for browner, more flavorful results with little added seasoning. Even if you live in a cold climate, outdoor grilling may be possible even in cooler weather. When grilling, experiment with different types of wood chips, like apple or hickory. Use hickory chips to add a delectable baconlike aroma and taste to chicken, even skinless.
- Use top quality foods, such as fresh, native produce, which are more flavorful and can stand on their own without high-fat additives.
- Acid flavors add interest to dishes and help compensate for a lack of salt. Freshly squeezed lemon juice is a good all-around seasoning. Also good are flavorful vinegars, such as Balsamic or herb vinegar. If you like sweet and tangy flavors, Balsamic vinegar makes a terrific salad dressing.
- Fresh garlic, ginger, black pepper, or chili pepper enliven dishes while keeping them low-salt.
- Fresh herbs are great for adding flavor, especially dill, thyme, rosemary, chives, oregano, and basil. You can grow these yourself in the summer outside. If you live in a cold climate, many herbs can be grown indoors on your windowsill. Add a potted rosemary bush for a year-round indoor herb garden. Generally, the more you use an herb plant, the thicker and bushier it grows, so even a few plants can provide a bountiful harvest for your kitchen.

What You Can Do: Treat yourself to a low-fat cookbook. Check the "Resources" section of this book for some excellent suggestions.

#28

Bake a Delicious Dessert!

Are we kidding? Doesn't being heart-healthy mean you have to give up desserts for good? Actually, since both of us authors have sweet tooths, we couldn't imagine such a thing.

It's possible to bake both sweet and heart-healthy, says Andrea Vegh Dunn, a registered dietitian from the Cleveland Clinic Foundation. What you need to learn to do is substitute and modify your current recipes. Here's an example.

Remember the carrot cake with the cream cheese frosting you've always loved? Rich, moist, and tasty—and also half your fat budget for the day! Although carrot cake may sound "healthy," a typical serving contains 32 grams of fat and a whopping 560 calories.

Want to still have your cake and be good to your heart, too? Substitute the oil with applesauce, and use fat-free substitutes for the eggs. Instead of the sticky-sweet frosting, dust the cooled cake with confectioners' sugar before serving. You'll eliminate all the fat, yet still have that moist, rich dessert you can easily work into your heart-healthy lifestyle—with only 262 calories per serving.

Try this modified carrot cake:

2 cups flour
1/2 cup sugar
1 tablespoon ground
cinnamon
1/2 teaspoon ginger
2 teaspoons baking soda
dash of salt

1 cup applesauce
1 (15-ounce) can crushed
pineapple, with syrup
2 cups lightly packed shredded carrots
1/2 cup fat-free egg substitute
1 teaspoon vanilla
1 cup golden raisins

Spray a cholesterol-free vegetable oil cooking spray on a 9-inch by 13-inch pan. Lightly dust with flour. Combine the dry ingredients in a large bowl. Stir in the remaining ingredients until well-mixed. Pour into the prepared pan. Bake at 350 degrees for 40 to 45 minutes. When cool, refrigerate 24 to 48 hours. Before serving, sprinkle lightly with confectioners' sugar. Makes 12 servings.

Here are Andrea Vegh Dunn's tips on modifying any recipe so you can create your own heart-healthy desserts. These alternatives work well not only in baking, but in making other dishes as well.

LOW-FAT SUBSTITUTIONS:
A CHANGE FOR THE BETTER

To replace	Substitute	Savings in calories/fat
1 whole egg	2 egg whites or 1/4 cup egg substitute	35 calories 5 grams fat
Whole milk	Skim milk, evaporated skim milk diluted with equal amounts of water, or reconstituted nonfat dry milk	Per cup (if using skim milk) 60 calories 8 grams of fat per cup
Cream or half & half	Undiluted evaporated skim milk or nonfat dry milk mixed double or triple strength	Per 1/4 cup (if using evaporated skim milk) 67 calories 11 grams of fat
Sour cream	Nonfat sour cream alternative or plain nonfat yogurt. If substituting the yogurt in a casserole or meat dish, add 1 t. cornstarch per cup yogurt to prevent curdling.	Per 1/4 cup 90 calories 12 grams of fat
Cream cheese	Dry curd low-fat cottage cheese blended with plain nonfat yogurt or skim milk to reach the consistency of cream cheese OR Line a sieve with cheesecloth or a coffee filter and place over an open container. Pour plain nonfat yogurt into the sieve. Cover and refrigerate overnight or longer until the consistency of cream cheese.	Per ounce 60 calories 9 grams of fat

Source: *Heartline*

She notes that you may find the new recipe is less moist than the original. Depending on the recipe, you can add applesauce, cut-up fruit, or nonfat yogurt to reduce this problem.

Shaving fat grams can make a big difference. For example, the average American eats sixteen pounds of ice cream a year. If you chose a nonfat frozen dessert rather than a premium high-fat ice cream, you'll be saving up to 1,000 grams of fat, or 9,000 calories a year. That 9,000 calories could translate to almost three pounds on your hips. So you really can have your cake and eat it too!

What You Can Do: Review your favorite recipes to see how you can modify them. Once that's done, cook up your favorite, then write it down and don't misplace it. Check the "Resources" section for a list of books that make low-fat cooking easy and delicious.

#29

DINE OUT RIGHT

We don't know about you, but ordering "scrod, plain with no butter" has never turned us on. You don't have to resort to such dining practices either. Here are some tips which will help you dine "heart-smart" while you *enjoy* dining out.

Our most important advice is to plan ahead. Nowadays, more and more restaurants are adding "healthy choices," like seafood, pasta, and salads to their menu. In fact, some restaurants offer entire "heart-healthy" menus. But you won't be able to take advantage of this if, at mealtime, you find yourself stranded with only the local rib-joint nearby.

Read restaurant advertisements and keep an eye out for menus touting "seasonal" dishes. Often, this connotes a chef who loves to use fresh herbs, greens, and other native veggies. This makes not only for delicious dining but often heart-healthy eating; these chefs don't like to obscure the flavor of these foods with rich, heavy sauces.

If you don't see any healthy choices which appeal to you on the menu, discuss this problem with your server. The chef may be able to substitute a simple tomato sauce for a cream-ladened pasta dish, for example. Request your entrées served with the sauce or gravy on the side. Spinach salad may be available without bacon. Often, substitutions can be made on short notice. This is not, though, generally true of very fancy restaurants which offer dishes made from precise, multi-ingredient recipes. But such eateries usually offer one or two lighter, and equally delicious specialties.

Don't starve yourself. There are plenty of filling choices on almost any menu. If you're really hungry, order a double salad, instead of filling up on buttered bread. Opt for restaurants that feature really good salads, not just a sorry collection of limp lettuce.

Sometimes, an entire dinner may be too much, especially if you're a light eater (or on your way to becoming one). You may find the appetizer portion, along with a salad and roll, to be the perfect amount. Many restaurants do not mind you ordering this way. You can specify that your food come when your dinner companions' entrées arrive. Check the menu, though, as some restaurants do require you order a minimum dollar requirement.

Don't hesitate to ask for a doggie bag. It's being done even in the ritziest of places. If the weather is warm, though, watch out for spoilage.

Beware of alcohol. It's always tempting to order a cocktail or glass of wine beforehand, but as we've noted, alcohol is fattening. What's more, alcohol can dissolve your resolve to eat right. If you want a glass of wine, make it last by ordering club soda as well, and creating a wine spritzer. Alcohol-free frozen drinks look and taste like the real thing. Alcohol-free beer is also an option. You're still consuming calories, but you'll keep your resolve.

Come meal's end, ignore the rich choices on the dessert tray. Many restaurants now offer fresh fruit, sorbet, or frozen low-fat yogurt. If you absolutely must have that sinful, restaurant dessert, consider making a withdrawal on your "fat budget." As we noted in the section on "Fat Banking," sometimes you just can't resist temptation. If that's how you feel, order the treat and enjoy it.

What You Can Do:
- Keep a file of those restaurants that feature heart-healthy dishes. That way, if you're dining out, or asked for a recommendation, you'll be assured of delicious foods you can enjoy.
- Be on the prowl for new restaurants. Read restaurant reviews, and take note when "light" or "healthy" dining is featured, or look for descriptions of dishes which feature fresh vegetables or fish instead of relying on butter and cream sauces.
- Buy a fat-gram counter which specializes in dining out. Check the "Resources" section.

#30

Have a Drink

A few years ago, alcohol made headlines when studies were released showing that drinking may actually be good for the heart. The media, along with liquor stores, jumped on the bandwagon. But before you take that drink, here are some facts to consider.

The studies we mentioned showed that moderate alcohol consumption may be good for your heart because it increases the level of HDL, the so-called "good" type of cholesterol in your blood.

When considering these studies, you must keep in mind that researchers evaluated the effects of moderate drinking. This is a drinking level strictly defined as one or two drinks a day, a standard drink being 12 ounces of beer, 4 ounces of wine, or 1.5 ounces of 80-proof spirit. For women, one drink a day is considered "moderate" because of their lesser body weight and differences in the way females metabolize alcohol.

For some people with heart disease, though, any alcohol

at all may be dangerous. For example, if you have high blood pressure, alcohol can raise it further. Some research has shown that drinking more than a moderate amount can cause a heart ailment resulting in heart dilation and weakness. Some studies in women have linked even a moderate amount of alcohol to an increased risk of breast cancer.

If you do not customarily drink, we suggest you not consider your heart as a reason to start. There are better ways, such as smart eating and exercise, to improve the health of your heart. On the other hand, if you are accustomed to an occasional, or even a daily, alcoholic drink, and your doctor has no objection, then let us be the first to join you in a toast.

What You Can Do:
- Ask your doctor about whether alcohol is an indulgence you can enjoy and how much is safe for you.
- If you drink, do you know how much you actually consume? Sometimes, we think we are heavier or lighter drinkers than we actually are. Keep track of how much alcohol you are consuming (both by number and strength of the drinks) to make certain it does not exceed that "moderate" amount.

CHAPTER SEVEN

GET ACTIVE

Many years ago, the treatment for people with heart problems consisted primarily of plenty of rest. Those with even the most minor of heart ailments were treated gingerly, and the idea that such people could participate in exercise would have been greeted with horror. But times change, and research has proved that, when it comes to treating heart problems, exercise may indeed be just what the doctor ordered. In fact, it is exercise which may prove to be one of the most powerful factors in returning you to a lifestyle which is not only as good as it was before you were diagnosed with heart disease, but better. Still, as a heart patient, there are some very important things you need to know. This information is covered in the next sections.

#31

CONSIDER EXERCISE
AS THERAPY, TOO

If you're like most people, you probably don't think of exercise as therapy. You may think of it as work or, if you enjoy it, as relaxation or a stress releaser. But exercise is, in fact, potent medicine for people with heart disease.

The good news is that you don't have to become Arnold Schwarzenegger or Jane Fonda to reap the benefits of exercise. Even a brisk daily walk can result in better cholesterol levels and lower blood pressure. Regular exercise can help prevent diabetes. If you are diabetic, exercise can help control your blood sugar levels. Studies also show that aerobic exercise improves your heart's capacity for work and, most importantly, can affect your metabolism, resulting in changes which can slow or even halt the development of atherosclerosis, the process which narrows your coronary arteries.

Exercise can also:

· Help you lose weight and keep it off.
· Help you quit smoking and stay off cigarettes.

- Tone your muscles.
- Help you sleep.
- Reduce stress.
- Enhance your self-esteem.

No matter what your age or physical condition, exercise can benefit you.

You may feel that you get enough exercise just working around the house or on your job. To benefit your heart, though, you need to participate in a regular exercise program.

As a heart patient, you need an individualized, safe exercise plan. The best way to do this is by participating in a cardiac rehabilitation program, which we discuss next. We are enthusiastic supporters of cardiac rehab, because we've seen the tremendous benefits these programs can bring.

If you do not have a cardiac rehabilitation program available to you, consider asking your doctor for a consultation with an exercise physiologist who can help you design your own program and give you tips about exercising safely. Sometimes, doctors are not up-to-date on the details of prescribing exercise and do not know how to best advise their patients to do it. They may simply advise you to "take a walk" when you could derive far greater benefits from an individualized exercise program. Or, they may not be familiar with studies that have shown that some patients who were never encouraged to exercise before, such as those with congestive heart failure, may indeed be able to exercise safely and improve their well-being.

What You Can Do: Read on! The next sections talk about cardiac rehab as well as different ways to become more active. If you do not have a cardiac rehabilitation program available to you, ask your doctor about arranging a consultation with an exercise physiologist who can help you design your own individualized program and give you—as a person with a heart problem—tips about safety and what to look for.

32

CONSIDER CARDIAC REHAB

If you're a heart attack survivor, you may have already participated in a cardiac rehabilitation ("cardiac rehab") program. But if you have not had a heart attack, you might be unaware that cardiac rehab benefits more than just heart attack victims. Indeed, almost anyone with heart disease can greatly benefit from participating in a well-run program.

The benefits afforded by cardiac rehab are often overlooked in today's cardiology world, which focuses on high-tech, "quick fix" treatments like balloon angioplasty or dramatic procedures like coronary bypass surgery. Cardiac rehab, though, can be an important adjunct for many and the primary therapy for some.

Cardiac rehab is a specially structured program of exercise, education, and psychological and social support designed to strengthen your heart's ability to perform exercise and return you to normalcy or better. A good cardiac rehab program provides you with more than just exercise; you benefit from the expertise of professionals with years of training and experience working with people who face the very same problems you face. You also make new friends, friends who know what you are going through because they've been there.

In the past, cardiac rehab was considered mostly for heart attack victims. Since then, the number of patients who may benefit has broadened. If you have chest pain ("angina") from heart disease, physical conditioning can increase endurance and delay the onset of chest pain. If you've had a heart attack, cardiac rehabilitation of more than twelve weeks duration appears to reduce the likelihood of your dying, especially in the first year afterward. Such programs will also benefit you if you've had coronary bypass surgery or balloon angioplasty. Studies show you can experience a 50 to 90 percent improvement in your ability to exercise after four months in such a program. It also places you under the watchful eye of a professional who can help you detect problems if they occur. Cardiac rehab has even been shown to be beneficial for people with badly damaged heart muscles or heart failure, because it improves their capacity to perform their daily activities.

In addition, if you've been diagnosed with a cardiac problem, you may suddenly feel very fragile. A cardiac rehab program provides you with a safe environment in which you can improve your strength and endurance to a point you never expected to achieve. A good rehab program also provides a variety of regular educational sessions: lectures, group discussions, fireside chats, workshops, etc. They offer support for the lifestyle changes you must make, providing low-fat cooking sessions, tips on quitting smoking, and a place where you can deal with the emotional issues that accompany heart problems.

Cardiac rehab differs from a regular exercise program in that you follow an exercise program that is highly individualized for you and your heart is monitored as you exercise. The pace is increased gradually, and modified according to your individual needs. The program may take place at a hospital, YMCA, or community gym. Any setting is fine, but you should make certain the program conforms to guidelines of the American Heart Association, the American College of Cardiology, and the American Association of Cardiovascular and Pulmonary Rehabilitation.

Unfortunately, women are less likely to join these programs and more likely to drop out. Some older women do not drive and find transportation an obstacle. Also, women sometimes tend to place their health on a lower priority and don't want to "inconvenience" anyone. So, if you're a woman, persevere, and find a program which is convenient and comfortable for you.

Remember, even if you had your heart attack or surgery years ago, it's not too late to join a cardiac rehab program. Such a program can improve your health, increase your knowledge and your sense of well-being, and help you meet new friends. Cardiac rehab can be a major ally in your fight to conquer heart disease.

What You Can Do:
- Ask your doctor if you are a candidate for cardiac rehabilitation.
- Explore the cardiac rehabilitation programs in your area. If you are a woman you may feel more comfortable if other women are in the program as well. Since women are less likely to be in cardiac rehab programs, you may have to check out a few to find the right program for you.

Once you find a program, check to make certain it meets these qualifications:

- Ask whether it conforms to guidelines of the American Heart Association, the American College of Cardiology, and the American Association of Cardiovascular and Pulmonary Rehabilitation.
- Is the program supervised by a cardiologist or otherwise qualified physician?
- Is there a qualified nurse or someone else with training *and* certification on hand at all times to handle medical emergencies?
- Do the exercise instructors have a college degree in physical fitness or a related field and have additional training in cardiac rehabilitation?

33

Get on Target

Before you embark on an exercise program there are two essential musts: The first is that you must get your doctor's clearance before you start. We know we keep saying this, but it's very important.

The second important thing is that you need to know your target heart rate to get the most you can from aerobic exercise, whether you are doing it as part of a cardiac rehabilitation program or part of an exercise program approved by your doctor. This knowledge both ensures you will be exercising vigorously enough to strengthen your cardiovascular system while at the same time ensuring that you will not overwork your heart.

Some people mistakenly think that if pushing your heart rate to its target rate is good, pushing it higher is even better. This is not true. If your heart rate goes up too high, this indicates that instead of exercising aerobically, which strengthens your cardiovascular system, you're exercising anaerobically, which means you're working too hard. To reap the benefits of aerobic exercise, you must stay within your target heart range.

To find your target heart range subtract your age from 220. Then, multiply that figure by 0.60 and 0.80. That figure will give you a heart rate value if you are working at 60 to 80 percent of maximum, which is considered a good level for cardiac conditioning. For example, if you are forty, your maximum heart rate should be about 180 (220–40) beats per minute. Your 60 to 80 percent target range is 108 (180 × .6) to 144 (180 × .8) beats per minute. Often, when doing aerobics, the instructor will have you take a ten-second measurement. Dividing by 6, this means your target heart rate should fall between 18 and 24 beats for a ten-second count. If it is higher than that, don't stop abruptly, but slow down. We have various pulse points on our bodies; two convenient places the pulse can be found are at the wrist and at the neck.

By the way, if you are in a cardiac rehab program and were tested for exercise capability, your heart rate may differ from those you derive from the above calculations. Use the target heart rate you were given in your program, since the rate is specific to your body.

When you are exercising, if you find your pulse rate is running too high, slow down the vigorousness of the activity a bit. If you are in an exercise class, for example, march in place. If your pulse rate is too low, put a little more intensity into your activities. If you are in an aerobics class, raising your arms up and down over shoulder level will generally raise your heart rate.

There is another easy way to test the intensity of your activity, especially if you and a friend are walking or using a treadmill or stationary bike. This is called the "Talk Test." If you can talk to your partner easily, your level of activity is probably below 80 percent of your maximum exercise capacity.

Regardless of your heart rate, if the exercise feels too strenuous, or if you begin to suffer from chest pain or other cardiac symptoms, stop! When you stop exercising, if you're still winded after ten minutes, or still tired after an hour, you're overdoing it. Contact your doctor if exercising brings on difficulty breathing, faintness, dizziness, nausea, confusion, chest pain, extreme fatigue, or leg pain.

Exercising right can bring you great benefits, so follow the few essential rules we outline and you will be exercising not only effectively, but safely as well.

What You Can Do: Practice finding your heart rate. See how your rate fluctuates when you do different types of exercise. Take it easy getting started. If you experience any symptoms such as chest pain, shortness of breath, dizziness, or undue fatigue, be sure to consult your doctor before exercising *any* further.

#34

TAKE A WALK (OR RUN)

If you really want to help your heart, forget joining that fancy health club or expensive gym and just start walking. Sounds simple, doesn't it? Studies show that walking is one of the best things you can do for your heart. Experts now say a brisk walk three times a week affords the same type of cardiovascular benefits once associated with more strenuous activities such as running and jogging.

Walking is a great exercise, and all you really need is a pair of well-fitting walking shoes. Invest in earphones and a Walkman, and you can enjoy tape-recorded music or even books while you walk (but watch carefully for vehicles since your hearing will be affected!). You can walk with a friend, or you can walk alone. If you live in a climate where it is sometimes too cold or rainy, and you want to walk, consider a large enclosed shopping mall. A mall is a good place to walk, and many malls have organized walking clubs. The possibilities are endless!

As with any other form of exercise, you should discuss

beginning a walking program with your doctor. Gradually build up the amounts of time you walk. Monitor your heart rate, especially when you're walking uphill.

How can you tell if you're walking at a safe pace? Monitor yourself by finding your target heart rate or employ the "Talk Test," discussed on page 124. Contact your doctor if you experience chest pain, shortness of breath, or other heart-related symptoms.

Even though walking does not involve an outlay of expensive equipment, put some money into your feet. Once upon a time, sneakers were the only "athletic shoes" available. But the sneaker has grown up, and scientifically sound exercise shoes are now available for walking or jogging. It's also important to dress for the elements. Several light layers of clothing are better than a single one. Also, don't walk outside if it's too cold or too hot; find a climate-controlled indoor location.

Set goals as you gradually increase your pace. Often, charity organizations sponsor walk-a-thons to promote worthy causes. Each October, the American Heart Association sponsors a nationwide five-mile walk-a-thon. You might find such an activity rewarding. Just make certain that you have conditioned yourself so that you can walk such a length comfortably and safely.

Walking can provide you with a great cardiovascular activity, but, as you become accustomed to walking longer and longer distances, you may be tempted to jog. Jogging can benefit your heart as well. Remember, though, to check with your doctor first. Once you've gotten clearance, here are some jogging tips.

To go from walking to running, you might start out by alternating walking with running. For example, if you are on a track, try running half a lap, then resume your walking pace. If you are walking over several blocks, alternate a block of walking with a block of running. Increase very gradually and, before you know it, you may be out jogging or running instead of walking. But again, be sure to monitor your heart rate and notify your doctor if you experience possible heart-related symptoms.

Beware of hard surfaces. Running on a softer, grassy surface will be softer on your ankles and knees and help you avoid injury. Once you are accustomed to running, try doing it on an uneven surface. This forces you to lift your legs higher, helps your balance, and strengthens your ankles. But be careful and watch out for holes and irregularities in the turf. Running injuries are a common occurrence.

Begin each jogging session with a warm-up. This could include a period of stretching exercises followed by a period of walking, before you begin to run. After your run, perform a "cool down" period similar to the warm-up.

What You Can Do:
- Invite your spouse, or a friend, to be your "walking partner." You may be surprised to find out how eager people are to join you.
- Contact your local affiliate of the American Heart Association for free pamphlets on walking and running.

#35

GET IN THE SWIM

Swimming can be as beneficial to your heart as other forms of exercise and many people find it more fun. Thanks to the buoyancy provided by the water, people with arthritis or joint problems can get an aerobic workout by swimming. But most people swim simply because they like it.

If you're considering swimming, here are some tips offered by Lynn Luthern, an exercise physiologist with the Cleveland Clinic Foundation's cardiac rehabilitation program, as well as advice from the American Heart Association on how to get started.

- As with other exercise programs, you must check with your doctor first. Being horizontal in the water shifts blood to the central part of the circulation (heart and lungs) so if your heart is badly damaged or you have lung problems, your doctor may suggest another form of exercise.
- Be careful you don't overexert yourself when swimming. When you are doing exercises out of the water, it's easier to

gauge what your level of exertion is. However, your perceptions may not be as accurate in the water. You may be swimming at what you think is a comfortable rate but you may actually be working at a much higher intensity.

• Indoor pools are preferable to swimming in an ocean or lake, which can turn out to be more taxing due to colder temperatures, currents, waves, or wind. The water should be warm (82–90 degrees) which, unfortunately, is warmer than the temperature of most pools in health clubs and community centers. So you may have to shop around to find a pool which is warm enough. Some health clubs, YMCAs, and YWCAs have physical-therapy programs which offer a warmer pool.

• Make sure there is a lifeguard or instructor on hand at all times.

• If you are not accustomed to exercising, consider joining a cardiac rehabilitation program, where you can learn how to determine your target heart rate and how to properly pace yourself. Tell the instructor you intend to swim so you can learn your ideal heart rate while swimming.

• As you begin, go easy on yourself. Begin with a half lap or as many laps as you can, even if it's only one or two. Increase the number of laps gradually.

• Begin each swimming session with ten to fifteen minutes of stretching exercises outside the pool. Start with a few slow laps to accustom yourself to the water. End each session the same way: with two slow laps to reduce your heart rate, and some stretching exercises after you emerge from the pool. This will relax your muscles and keep them from tightening later on.

Some pools offer water exercise classes. These can range from classes offering easy stretches to intensive cardiovascular workouts. Be sure you choose the right level for you.

What You Can Do:
- Get your doctor's okay before you begin a swimming program.
- If your swimming skills are rusty, consider a few lessons. This can help you get more enjoyment out of the sport.

36

CONSIDER PUMPING IRON

Strength training, which sometimes involves lifting weights and is also known as strength-resistance training, can be a boon for getting into better shape than you ever thought imaginable, even in the days when you did not have heart disease.

You may have never considered working out with strength-training equipment. Consider it! Although aerobic exercise strengthens the cardiovascular system, it does not, by itself, help prevent osteoporosis, the so-called "brittle bone" disease which affects many older women. This is where strength-training comes in: Not only will it help prevent osteoporosis, it will also tone you and help you look great!

Before you hit the barbells, though, here are "do's and don't's" to keep in mind from Gordon Blackburn, Ph.D., of the Cleveland Clinic Foundation's cardiac rehabilitation program.

If you are considering weight-training, get your doctor's

permission. If you have congestive heart failure, uncontrolled high blood pressure, heart valve problems, severe coronary artery disease, or heart rhythm problems, training with weights is not usually recommended.

When you undertake strength-resistance training, the program should be individualized based on your needs, interests, and medical condition.

Most people think of weight training as "pumping iron," but your own body weight may provide enough resistance for certain exercises. For example, leg lifts use the weight of the foot and lower leg as they are lifted against gravity as resistance. You can add ankle weights as you progress.

Colorful tubing or rubber bands, which are large strips of rubber, are also used for another form of strength-resistance exercising. The strips can be looped between your legs or arms or between your limb and a doorknob while exercising, providing added resistance. The amount of resistance can vary, depending on the size of the band and the degree of stretch in the rubber band.

For the more advanced, free weights can be used. This category includes dumbbells, barbells, or even common household items like soup cans. Proper form when using weights is essential, so it greatly helps to consult a qualified instructor to show you how to use them, and to review your form. Many health clubs and gyms also feature resistance machines that work specific sets of muscles. These machines provide an added safety feature over free weights, especially at heavier weights, because the machine ultimately supports the weight if you can't lift it.

For best results, you should do resistance exercises from three to five times weekly. Always monitor your heart rate. Your exercise heart rate should be lower during resistance training than during aerobic exercise. Your trainer can help you determine a good heart-rate level for you. Remember, stop exercising immediately if you feel any chest discomfort, palpitations, lightheadedness, or shortness of breath.

Strength-resistance training is not, however, a substitute for aerobic exercise. It will not strengthen your cardiovascular system. When used together with aerobic exercise, it can provide a more well-rounded conditioning program.

What You Can Do: After you get your doctor's okay, consult an exercise expert for instruction. A cardiac rehabilitation program would be the perfect place to find a knowledgeable and qualified trainer. If this consultation is part of your rehabilitation program, the cost may even be covered by your insurance.

#37

"Sneak In" Even More Physical Activity

The old motto "no pain, no gain" is happily now in the garbage can. The good news is that moderate exercise is now in vogue, thanks to recommendations released in 1993 by the Centers for Disease Control and Prevention. According to these recommendations, each of us "should accumulate thirty minutes or more of moderate-intensity physical activity" at least five days a week.

What's the big news in that? The word "accumulate"! Formerly, the recommendations held that you had to perform at least twenty to thirty minutes of continuous aerobic activity to strengthen your cardiovascular system. But being able to "accumulate" exercise and spread it throughout the day can make it all the more easy to "sneak in" more physical activity into your daily life.

- At home, answer the phone in the room farthest away from you.
- At work, take a walking break instead of a coffee break.

Take a brisk walk around the floor or building. And use the stairs, of course, instead of the elevator.

- If you're in a car pool, have the driver pick you up or drop you off several blocks from home or work. Make certain, of course, that you're left off in a safe area. Perhaps you and a fellow worker can walk partway home together.
- Go window shopping. Leave your wallet at home, though, or this could become an expensive habit.
- Walk the family dog. No dog? Borrow your neighbor's.
- Do your errands on foot. For instance, drive partway to the post office and walk the rest of the way when you need stamps. Walk to the store instead of sending your kids.
- Join a bowling league or other organized sports activity.
- When shopping at the mall, park as far away as safely possible and walk to the stores. Remember, though, safety first!
- If you work in a high rise, stop the elevator two or three stops before your stop and take the stairs the rest of the way.
- When it comes to stairs, only take an elevator if you're going up more than one floor, or down two.
- Live in an apartment? Bring your trash to the utility room daily instead of using the chute (watch those steps, though, when carrying anything).
- Take a ten to fifteen minute walk after dinner. Enjoy the sunset. This is a romantic activity with a companion but also relaxing when you're alone.

What You Can Do: Think of more ways you can "sneak in" exercise. Then do them!

CHAPTER EIGHT

STRESS AND YOUR HEART

If you look at any bookstore's psychology or self-help sections, you'll find no shortage of books on the dangers of "killer" stress. Indeed, stress has been blamed for numerous maladies, from headaches to heart attacks. If you've suffered a heart attack, plenty of people have probably told you that you have to do something about your stress. But what? Stress is a part of daily life. Some people appear to thrive on stress, while for others it proves to be their psychological undoing.

What's the story about stress when it comes to your heart? The following sections explore what is known about stress, how to identify the stressors in your life, and how to keep stress within manageable limits.

#38

INVENTORY YOUR STRESS

Although experts agree that risk factors such as smoking and obesity can cause heart disease, there is no such consensus about the role of stress. Some studies link stress with heart disease, others do not.

We believe that reducing unhealthy stress can help you fight heart disease. Eventually, a direct link may be proven. But in the meantime, stress clearly contributes to such unhealthy practices as eating too much, abusing alcohol, and smoking. All of these can lead to damage of your heart.

The dictionary defines stress as "any interference that disturbs a person's healthy mental and physical well-being." When we are under stress, our autonomic nervous system responds by increasing production of hormones that increase our heart rate, raise our blood pressure, and speed our metabolism.

Some researchers believe this release of hormones contributes to the development of heart disease by adversely affecting your cholesterol profile. This theory holds that these hormones can cause the so-called "bad" LDL-cholesterol to circulate longer in your bloodstream.

Stress is a complicated and very individual issue. First of all, what's bad stress for one person may be enjoyably exciting for another. For example, some people, when called to speak in a group, undergo horrible symptoms of stage fright. Others, though, enjoy a little "zip" of adrenaline.

But if you're under so much pressure you feel you can never catch up, if you suffer from such stress-induced symptoms as migraine headaches, or if you're preoccupied with constant worrying, then you don't need to read a book to learn the effects of negative stress. You're living it!

However, changing habits, even ones resulting in negative stress, can be extremely difficult. Understanding stress can help you identify the sources in your life so you can make changes.

Both men and women are subjected to stress, although the different role each plays in society may result in different types of stress. The ways in which we've learned to think can also be stress-inducing.

For example, many people are prone to a "straitjacket" way of thinking, according to Michael G. McKee, Ph.D., head of the Cleveland Clinic Foundation's section of Biofeedback and Applied Psychophysiology. By this, he means that we tend to lock ourselves into psychological "straitjackets" by clinging to rules we may not consciously realize we follow. These messages we may tell ourselves include such edicts as "anything worth starting is worth finishing," or "if you can't do it well, it's not worth doing." So, we sometimes fail to give ourselves permission to give up a task, even when it's frustrating us.

Most women, and some men, are faced with stress from multiple roles. Years ago, a woman's role was spread out over her lifespan. She worked, then got married and stayed home until her youngest child entered school, and then perhaps returned to the workforce. Most women cannot afford this economic luxury today, and must frantically juggle their roles of housewife, mother, and consummate professional. Men, too, can be subject to changing societal expectations. They may be expected to play a greater role in raising children, but feel ill-equipped because they never saw their fathers in this role.

This is the age of the "sandwich generation." Women especially are often caught between the demands of raising children and coping with the needs of aging parents. At the age of seventy-two, when she expected to be taking it easier, Eleanor found herself suffering from increased chest pain. "I noticed my symptoms have gotten worse ever since my mother moved in with me," says Eleanor. Her mother is ninety-two!

Being diagnosed with heart disease can cause stress in itself. You may be afraid you can't do the things you used to do. You may be uncertain about how this disease will affect your job or your family.

While you can't eliminate stress completely, nor would you want to, you can learn to reduce it. In the coming sections, we'll share methods which have helped even the most hard-core stress addicts.

What You Can Do:
- Take a "stress inventory" of yourself. Do you have "straitjacket" ways of thinking? Are you part of the "sandwich generation"? Does your job give you stress or are you "stressed out" by visiting certain people?
- Map out a strategy about how to deal with it. If you're part of the "sandwich generation," for example, and caring for an elderly parent, seek out community services which can help.

#39

REDUCE
YOUR JOB
STRESS

When you are taking your stress inventory, you may find that your job crops up on the list. Many of us barter away our lives, working at jobs we dislike. Being diagnosed with heart disease, or suffering a cardiac crisis, can unleash dissatisfaction that has been just simmering below the surface.

After a dramatic personal event, such as a heart attack or diagnosis of heart disease, experts say that people should be cautious about making life-changing decisions. But sometimes waiting isn't feasible. Your job requirements may force you to contemplate change. For example, if your job involves physical labor, you may be transferred or you may decide you need a change. If just thinking about your job puts you under so much stress that you can feel it eating away at you, it might be wise to consider a change. But be certain you think it through.

Take George, for example. An executive in a large, well-known manufacturing company, George hated his job. "I always thought that selling ice cream would be a happy way to make a living," George said. So, he accepted early retirement from his company and bought a popular ice-cream shop franchise. Within six months, he was miserable. "I didn't realize that, unless I wanted to be in the shop constantly, I'd have to hire help to run it. The help I could afford were totally irresponsible. They wouldn't show up or they'd make mistakes and I'd have to run down to the shop at a moment's notice," says George. He also never realized how demanding the consuming public could be. Back to the corporate world he went.

Changing your job may not automatically change your personality. Witness Henry. Henry decided to take his cardiologist's advice to live a "less stressful" life to heart, and moved to the Virgin Islands! Before long, he realized that the little beachtown where he lived could use a jeep livery service. Henry started one. Then he realized a marina was needed. Henry started that too. Then a hotel. Before long, he owned half the town, and was as stressed out as before!

On the other hand, job changes can sometimes work out very well. Shirley was caught in what we've dubbed a "stress sandwich." She used to work on a factory production line, but had been promoted to supervisor. Although she welcomed the new job, and the raise, she suddenly found herself in the position of supervising all her friends and former coworkers on the line. They simmered with resentment. Her boss, of course, expected her to maintain high-pressure production quotas. "I was having nightmares about what to do," Shirley recalls. After her heart attack, she discussed her concerns with her manager. Thanks to a transfer, Shirley was able to keep her promotion, and her friends.

Evaluate your job. Look for changes you can make within your workplace. If your job is impossible, consider a change. But be certain your decisions are sound. Discuss them with your family, your doctor, and possibly a social worker, therapist, or vocational counselor. That way, you'll maximize the chances that the change will be a success.

What You Can Do:
- If you are considering a job change, do your homework. Talk to friends in the business you are considering and get the lowdown on the pros and the cons. Consider job counseling. Because of the current company trend of downsizing, job counselors are more accustomed to dealing with older people.
- Remember that working for yourself does not necessarily relieve stress. Heart disease may make you feel not only insecure about your health, but your finances as well. You may find yourself wondering if you have enough money set aside if other health problems arise, or you may find yourself thinking about early retirement. Before you invest your savings in a franchise or other business opportunity, check it out thoroughly with the Better Business Bureau, your state Consumer Protection Department, and other appropriate authorities.

#40

Evaluate Your Relationships

If you've been through a medical crisis, you may find yourself undergoing changes in how you feel about friends and family. A diagnosis of heart disease can cause some people to be aware that time is fleeting, and no one lives forever. You may find yourself wanting to spend more time with the people you treasure, and less with those you find irritating.

. If you've suffered a heart attack, or some other type of cardiac crisis, you may also find yourself reevaluating your relationships with family and friends. We like to think that serious illness, such as heart disease or a heart attack, will draw friends closer. Generally it does, but sometimes it doesn't. You may find your emotions shaky and your relationships with friends and loved ones frayed.

Especially after a cardiac crisis such as a heart attack, you may be puzzled by changes in your friends' attitudes. They may draw back a little, or be distant. Heart disease is a powerful reminder of mortality; your friends may not only be frightened for you, but for themselves as well. This is what happened to Ellen after she suffered a heart attack at the age of forty-five. "My friends seemed slightly different to me. Almost aloof, like they didn't know what to do or say," Ellen recalls. After talking with a counselor, Ellen realized that her friends were afraid. "They realized that if I could have a heart attack, anyone could," she said.

As a spouse often does, your friends may become overprotective, when you don't need such coddling at all. Just as you may be wondering whether you'll ever go hiking again, or dance until dawn, so are they. In time, these fears will fade, and your relationships should return to normal. Communication is important. Talk with your friends openly and honestly. They probably don't even realize how they are acting.

If you believe there are people that make your life intolerable, be aware that the stress of dealing with them may not be doing your heart good. This is not an excuse to seek out an immediate divorce. But a cardiac crisis often makes people reflective. If this sounds like you, it's important not to make snap decisions. How you feel now may be different from how you feel later on. If you feel this is indeed the time to make important changes in your life, consider seeing a counselor or therapist for an objective viewpoint and needed support.

This may also be a time to let go of past grudges. Practice forgiveness. Slights can turn into major offenses. Clinging to them can poison your emotional well-being. Find it in your heart to forgive.

What You Can Do:
- Consider the roles you play in the lives of your friends. Are they based on old, undesirable habits, like being your group's "champion" eater or "work horse"? Consider how you might change

these roles and what your friends' reactions might be. Discuss it with them.
- Consider the relationships you treasure. Are there old friends you have lost touch with? Are there friends whom you take for granted? This might be a good time to reestablish lost relationships and tell those you care for just how much you appreciate them.

#41

LEARN TO RELAX

"Reduce my stress? WHAT DO YOU MEAN, 'REDUCE MY STRESS'?" thundered Steve. The vessels in his neck throbbed at even the mildest suggestion that perhaps he might be just feeling a little stressed out.

Sometimes, even the topic of stress can, well, cause stress. This is because, too often, the person jumps to the conclusion that they need a total personality transplant. If you're bombastic, you're not going to be transformed overnight into blasé. But there are some techniques you can learn to reduce your stress.

The first step toward reducing your stress is finding out what causes it. This usually just involves paying attention to the things (or people), who trigger a stressed response in you. Sometimes, you can eliminate these causes. For example, if always arriving late leaves you in a tizzy, set the alarm earlier.

Michael G. McKee, Ph.D., an expert in stress management at the Cleveland Clinic, has some favored techniques for helping people relax.

He recommends stretching exercises and deep breathing as good ways to start relaxing. Here's a good relaxation exercise: Breathe in gently as you let your head drop back. Exhale as you let your head fall forward as far as it will go naturally and comfortably. Breathe deeply, with the diaphragm pushing down while your chest remains almost still. This type of breathing is central to relaxing. Once you become accustomed to it, you can use it as a secret weapon, employing it whenever you get into a stressful situation.

Systemic relaxation exercises include progressively relaxing and tensing the muscles in different muscle groups. There are many different ways to do this. Lie on the floor or sit comfortably in a chair. You can even practice this technique at your desk. Another technique is called focused imagery, which takes about fifteen minutes and involves focusing on a favorite image or sound. See our section, "Go to Arosa," for one way to accomplish this.

Some people get excited easily. An event that would mildly annoy some, like being cut-in-front-of in a grocery store, infuriates them. If you are like this, try a technique used by Lynda Powell, Ph.D., an epidemiologist at the Rush Presbyterian/St. Luke's Medical Center in Chicago. We call it "think like a fish." When you wake up each morning, think of yourself as a fish swimming peacefully in a beautiful stream. Suddenly a baited hook drops into your field of vision.

This "hook" could be a ringing phone, noisy children, the realization you've overslept, or some other annoyance of daily life. If you snap at that bait, you're more likely to snap up subsequent hooks and spend the whole day feeling upset, angry, and simmering with harmful hostility. If, on the other hand, you learn to think of such annoyances as hooks, you'll be more inclined to let them glide by. Sounds simple, doesn't it? But it works!

If you are still unable to relax after using these techniques, you might consider biofeedback training. Biofeedback training involves learning how to react properly to stressful situations. With biofeedback training, a variety of safe, noninvasive machines are used to measure what happens to your body under stress. Muscle tension, body temperature, skin response, and heart rate can be measured. You learn what a body part feels like when its tense and when it's relaxed. Over time, you learn how to achieve a calm response in situations which previously caused anxiety.

If you find others in your family are under stress, consider joining a stress-reducing program together. But remember, what works for one person does not necessarily work for another.

What You Can Do: Try the stress-reducing exercises in this book. If they work, practice them regularly. Check out the books on this topic listed in our "Resources" section. If stress continues to be a problem for you, explore such resources as your local hospital or community college to find out about stress management classes.

#42

LET'S BE FRENCH!

A few years ago, the "French Paradox" hit the media and the cardiology world hasn't been the same since. If you saw the CBS show "60 Minutes," or other media accounts, you're probably aware of this supposed contradiction. The "French Paradox" refers to the fact that the French traditionally eat high-fat food, but they have a much lower rate of heart disease than do Americans.

Bear in mind that the French lead a much different lifestyle than we do. If you adopt some aspects of the French way of life (not necessarily with all the rich food, though), you can help your heart.

Typically, the French do not rush out for "power breakfasts," or "power lunches," for that matter. The concept is quite unknown. Their pace of life is far more leisurely.

In fact, investigators at Boston University and the Centre de Recherches Foch, Paris, point out this difference in eating habits. The French consume more than half of their daily calories at midday, typically waiting five or more hours before their next meal. This pattern may have a beneficial effect on lipid (fat) metabolism. They also note that the French snack less, getting only 8 percent of their daily calories from snacks, while Americans, on the other hand, get as many as *22 percent of their daily calories from snacking.*

In the United States, there's an emphasis on speed. Some restaurants offer such specials as a "ten-minute guarantee," promising that if your meal isn't in front of you that quickly, it's free. Even that isn't fast enough for many of us. Thanks to the portable telephones and computers, business is conducted anywhere, all the time, including while we eat. In France, "cutting a deal" during a meal would be considered truly gauche!

What is generally missing in France is a concept that, if anything, defines us in the United States. That concept of "time urgency." Yet it is "time urgency" that many stress experts believe contributes to heart disease.

Enthusiasts of the "French Paradox" note that the French customarily drink wine, especially red wine, with their meals. We've written of the benefits of alcohol and the heart. It's worth noting, though, that even those who enthusiastically point to the "French Paradox" are not advocating drinking alcohol to excess.

Another major difference between us and the French is our "couch potato" lifestyle. It's not uncommon for French people to walk or bicycle to work. This type of exercise can add up. This is another reason why the "French Paradox" may not be such a paradox after all.

What You Can Do: When it comes to combining exercise and a leisurely, stress-free lifestyle, by all means, "let's be French."

#43

Go to Arosa (or Someplace Else Wonderful!)

Visualization is a technique where you learn to fine-tune your imagination to transport yourself to a pleasurable time or place. This can be wonderfully relaxing.

We discovered the visualization technique several years ago from Maurice, a French cousin. In his honor, we've named it "Going to Arosa," but you can, of course, pick the place which is special to you.

Maurice, a delightful gentleman, was a busy commercial contractor. For years, he worked from 7 A.M. to noon, walked home, and then enjoyed a leisurely lunch. After lunch, he would go out onto his balcony, close his eyes, and bask in the sun. When asked what he was thinking about, he replied, "I'm going to Arosa."

Arosa, it turns out, is a small, picturesque town in Switzerland, and Maurice's favorite vacation spot. He used to go there every year to ski. In Arosa, he stayed in a chalet which also had a balcony. Each day, after lunch, he would go sit out on the balcony and watch the skiers. So, said Maurice, "what

I do here everyday is go on my balcony, sit in the sun, close my eyes, and watch the skiers in my mind." After his brief, special "visit" to Switzerland, he would return to work refreshed.

It would amuse Maurice to learn that he is practicing a technique formally known as "visualization." This form of meditation requires no special skill, just an ability to visualize a place you enjoy, a place where you are free from stress, a place that brings a smile to your face. It takes only a few minutes to "go to Arosa," or whatever special place you want to go, every day. But we promise you, the journey is worthwhile. In fact, it gets better with practice.

What You Can Do: "Visualization" is considered by many a stress-relaxation technique that works. Give it a try. Pick your favorite destination and close your eyes. Voilà! You're there!

CHAPTER NINE

GET THE MOST
OUT OF LIFE

One of the biggest fears men and women with heart disease have is that they won't be able to do what they did before. But what we have found is that many people can not only do what they did before, they go on to do much more. For many people, heart disease is not the "end of the line" but a positive beginning. What follows are some suggestions on how to further enrich your life.

By the way, this book does not have an Epilogue. You may be coming to the end of this book, but you are certainly not coming to the end of your personal goals in living with heart disease. After all, we've presented you with 50 essential things you can do. But we have absolutely no doubt that, as you continue your reading, work with your doctor, and talk with your friends at your local "heart club" you'll come up with lots more.

#44

Enjoy Sex

Sexual relations are a natural part of adult life, and certainly not a pleasure you must bid "farewell" to if you have been diagnosed with heart disease or if you've suffered a heart attack. Unfortunately, though, people sometimes think that way, either out of uncertainty, lack of knowledge, or simply, fear.

Take Jerry, for example. At the age of sixty-seven, he was in a hospital cardiac care ward, having just undergone a coronary bypass operation, when he sent for his doctor. "What's the matter? I understand you're doing fine," the doctor said. Jerry, though, was despondent. "You don't understand. I've just gotten married! How am I going to keep up with my young bride?" Jerry said, referring to his new fifty-five-year-old wife. When assured his sex life was definitely not over, Jerry perked up considerably.

If you were having sexual problems before, a diagnosis of heart disease is not going to help matters any. Sadly, either patient or partner may embrace a heart problem as an excuse to forestall sex not temporarily, but permanently. Lack of sexual desire may also reflect another problem such as depression.

It doesn't have to be that way. The key to a good sexual relationship is the same as the key to any other good relationship: communication. The couple who is accustomed to discussing their problems frankly can often find it easy to iron out differences in the sexual arena once the topic is broached.

Honest communication with your doctor is also essential. But sex can be a difficult topic to bring up in the doctor's office. Even if the subject of sex leaves you tongue-tied or blushing, give it a try. After a few words, your doctor should be able to pick up the conversational ball. If you're female, and your doctor is male, you might feel more comfortable discussing the problem with a female doctor or nurse. Likewise, if your doctor is female, and you're male, you might feel more comfortable talking to a male health professional, if there is one in the office.

Unfortunately, though, some doctors are not very good at discussing sex. If this is the case, it often helps to be as specific as possible about your concern. According to Leslie R. Schover, Ph.D., who is a member of the Cleveland Clinic Foundation's Center for Sexual Function, men with heart disease sometimes experience difficulty in achieving and maintaining an erection, and this problem can worsen after a heart attack. However, psychological, medical, and surgical treatments for this problem are available.

The most common problem women experience after a heart attack or heart surgery is loss of sexual desire. Dr. Schover attributes this to depression, as heart patients are often naturally depressed about their health. Women also tend to fear that they've become less attractive, possibly due to a surgical scar. Older women also commonly experience vaginal dryness, which can make intercourse uncomfortable and even painful. This problem may be due to the decrease in estrogen that accompanies menopause. In this case, a good vaginal lubricant may be effective, or you might want to consider hormone replacement therapy (see page 66). For both men and women, some cardiovascular drugs can inhibit sexual desire.

If your doctor cannot supply you with the information you need, don't suffer in silence. Consider asking your doctor for a referral. If you're a male, consider consulting a urologist trained to deal with sexual problems. If you're female, your gynecologist may be quite helpful. Sometimes, discussing your problem with a mental health professional who specializes in sexual problems can be useful. Also, check the "Resources" section for books dealing with the subject of human sexuality.

One of the biggest fears experienced by both men and women is the worry that sexual excitement will lead to a heart attack or another complication, like "tearing my stitches" if you've undergone coronary bypass surgery. Happily, this fear simply is not grounded in fact. If you are able to climb a flight of stairs without becoming short of breath or experiencing chest pain (this is far less exertion than the amount you usually will achieve if you follow the "essential" exercise steps outlined in this book), you should be able to resume passive sex with your usual partner with safety. If you are planning to be the active partner, or anticipate finding sex especially exciting (with a new partner, perhaps) being able to climb two flights of stairs without breathlessness or chest pain is the rule-of-thumb.

Also, consider switching your sexual encounter from night to mornings when you are more rested, and don't indulge in sex after eating a big meal or heavy drinking. If you experience cardiac symptoms such as angina, the chest pain that sometimes accompanies heart disease, during sex, discuss it with your doctor. You may be advised to take nitroglycerin before sex to lessen such symptoms.

Above all, be patient with yourself and your partner. Remember, a diminished sex drive is not unusual after a heart attack or heart surgery, and, with time, normalcy should return. If, however, you find this problem becoming cemented into a pattern, you should discuss it with your doctor.

Sex is a healthy, normal part of life, and an activity you should certainly not have to sacrifice to heart disease. In fact, if you follow the other essential steps in this book, like quitting smoking, losing weight, and improving your physical condition, you may find yourself enjoying sex more than you have in years!

> *What You Can Do:* If you have any concerns regarding sex, talk frankly to your doctor. If your doctor does not welcome such discussion, consider taking your concerns to another health professional. Also, check the "Resources" section for books dealing with sexuality.

#45

Deal With Depression

Suffering a heart attack, undergoing a cardiac crisis, or sometimes even simply being diagnosed with heart disease can trigger depression. Depression can not only endanger your emotional well-being, it can also endanger your health. Women with heart disease are so often found to be depressed that some consider it a risk factor for heart disease. But men are vulnerable to depression as well.

That depression may accompany heart disease is not surprising. After all, depression is related to the loss of self. Learning you have heart disease can lead to grieving; grieving for not only your heart but also your sense of self-esteem. You may also fear the future.

You may have absorbed the idea, years ago, that heart disease is a death sentence, and you probably believe that deep down. You may have a parent or sibling who died of heart disease, and fear you will suffer the same fate.

Being depressed can magnify your worries, and make it more difficult for you to take the steps needed to deal with heart disease. If you're a man, you may not want to admit you're scared or depressed. It's not "macho," after all. A woman may prefer to suffer silently, not wishing to worry her family.

In many cases, the depression may be transitory, and taking action, such as following the "Essential Things" outlined in this book will make you feel better. But if you do not feel the cloud of despair lifting, and if you have any of the following "danger" signs of depression, you should discuss this problem with your doctor immediately. Once, depression was seen as a sign of weakness, but that is no longer true today. It is now viewed as a biological illness that can be successfully treated.

Signs of depression include:

- Sleep and appetite disturbances.
- Feeling your life is hopeless and not worth living.
- Feelings of fatigue or agitation not related to your physical condition.
- Loss of interest in usual activities.
- Trouble concentrating or making decisions.
- Crying, especially spontaneous spells.
- Suicidal thoughts.

> *What You Can Do:* When you are in the midst of depression, it may seem impossible that you will ever feel better. Contact your doctor for help. Depression is treatable.

#46

LAUGH ONCE EACH DAY (AT LEAST!)

One of the best things you can do for your heart is enjoy a hearty laugh. Laughing not only lifts your spirits, it promotes good health as well. In his book *Anatomy of an Illness*, author Norman Cousins described how laughter helped him overcome his severe illness. At first, his views were treated skeptically, but eventually they achieved wide acceptance.

"You don't need to be a brain surgeon to know laughing makes you feel good," notes Izzy Gesell, of Northampton, Massachusetts, who writes and speaks on the health benefits of humor. "When you laugh, you exercise your lungs, your heart, and your diaphragm. It's also a terrific way to reduce stress, which can help lower blood pressure."

After all, when someone with a heart condition becomes upset sitting in a traffic jam, it builds tension and makes the heart work harder. "If you can laugh, put on Groucho glasses, or play with a toy, you can distract yourself from getting tied up in knots about something you can't do anything about," Gesell added.

You may be thinking that this is all well and good for people who walk around grinning, but what if you don't consider yourself naturally humorous? According to Gesell, a sense of humor, like other behaviors, can be learned.

He suggests keeping a humor diary, writing down every time you laugh, and what generated the response. "Write down the sorts of things that, while you're watching the news on TV, you might point out to your husband or wife and say, 'Isn't that funny' or 'Isn't that weird?' You'll soon discover that humor is all around you," he said.

It isn't only jokes that bring a smile to people's faces. Pay attention to the small things in life that make you smile. As adults, we're not trained to honor humor, so we let these moments escape. Says Gesell, "Set your mental channel to look for humor in your life. Write down the things that make you laugh or smile and pass them along to others."

Gesell believes in positive humor, not negative humor which separates people. He urges his clients to be playful. But the most important thing, he says, is "learn to laugh at yourself."

"Gently acknowledging our own flaws and foibles is the best way to begin expanding our sense of humor. *Learn to take your life seriously, but yourself lightly.*"

What You Can Do: The key is to "be prepared" so you can plan ahead for frustration and have some sure-fire humor "activators" close at hand. Here are some suggestions:

- Whenever you need the benefits of humor, stop what you're doing and smile. Either close your eyes and lift the corners of your mouth or go over to a mirror, force a smile, and hold it for fifteen seconds.
- Try to think of a joke or observation appropriate for the sit-

uation and tell it to yourself. Do this by looking for the incongruity in the situation.

- Make a collection of ten things that bring you pleasure. Examples are pictures of your kids or pets, a card or note of appreciation that you received, an award you received at some time in your life, or a note or picture of yourself doing an activity you enjoy. Keep a list with you.
- Find and display a picture of yourself smiling or laughing. This will provide a humor role model for you.
- Put together a personal Humor Maintenance Outfit (HMO). For example, Izzy carries with him a few things he finds funny: Groucho glasses, Silly Putty, Play-Doh, whistle, Koosh Ball, and a smattering of wind-up toys. You might want to include cartoons, fuzzy dice dangling from the dashboard; anything that makes you smile. Keep this in the car in the event you get stuck in a traffic jam, or in your drawer at work.
- Conduct a "Pleasure Hunt." Go through your drawers, photo albums, and closets. Get reacquainted with the wonderful things you've tucked away. Put some in your "HMO."

#47

TAKE A TRIP

When you're diagnosed with heart disease, or if you've had a heart attack, you may question whether you'll be able to do everything you're accustomed to. If traveling falls into that category, start packing. There's no quicker way to become imprisoned in your own home than avoiding travel. But, to be a savvy traveler, there are a few things to keep in mind.

Many people with heart problems worry about the possibility of an in-flight cardiac emergency, says Dr. Richard N. Matzen, an expert in aviation medicine at the Cleveland Clinic Foundation. Such emergencies do happen, but very infrequently. According to Dr. Matzen, one study found a rate of one in-flight emergency for every 39,600 passengers. Only 20 percent of these were cardiac related, making the ratio one in-flight cardiac emergency for each 198,000 travelers. If you take into consideration non-inflight emergencies, for example the people waiting in the terminal, the number of cardiac-related emergencies is 1 for every 500,000 passengers. These are very slim odds indeed.

You may be concerned about the effect of altitude and the decrease in oxygen pressure while in flight. Most people have no problem at altitudes below ten thousand feet. Modern passenger jets fly at far higher altitudes, but pressurized cabins maintain an artificial altitude of eight thousand to ten thousand feet or less, making air travel generally safe, even on most older planes.

So, air travel generally poses few risk for heart patients. In terms of safety, flying is safer than driving. However, flight creates conditions which make even supposedly healthy people vulnerable to problems. To decrease your risk during air travel:

- Discuss the upcoming trip with your physician in case there are any individual precautions you should take. This is particularly true if you've suffered a heart attack within the past few months or if you have congestive heart failure. But it's good advice for heart patients in general.
- Exercise daily to stay fit, in accordance with your physician's wishes, of course.
- People on longer flights have an increased probability of experiencing symptoms, although not necessarily serious ones. If you're contemplating a long trip, consider taking shorter "legs" of a flight with a stop between.
- Allow plenty of time to get to the airport so you don't need to rush, especially if you're carrying a bag.
- If you are carrying luggage, get a porter's help with your baggage or use a bag outfitted with wheels.
- If you experience any symptoms, report them to airport or airline personnel.
- Keep your medicines readily available.
- Keep a resumé of your medical history with you, and re-

quest a copy of your EKG from your doctor before traveling.

There is one thing for the savvy traveler to be on guard against, though, and that is what has been described as "Economy Class Syndrome." People are crammed increasingly closer together in planes, and their legs become cramped. This can result in the formation of venous blood clots, which can break loose and cause serious problems, possibly even sudden death. Even healthy people can experience "Economy Class Syndrome," but if you have a history of heart failure, leg injuries, varicose veins, are dehydrated, or are overweight, you are at greater risk. To avoid it, follow these steps:

- If you're not already taking aspirin, consult your doctor about the advisability of taking an aspirin a day just before, during, and a week after a trip. Aspirin reduces the risk of blood clot formation.
- Get advice from your doctor about the proper socks to wear and if therapeutic support hose are recommended for you.
- Avoid any garment that causes constriction from the groin to the ankle.
- Continually stretch and flex your legs and walk around as much as possible.
- If you are a large person, consider upgrading to business or first class.
- Drink a lot of nonalcoholic beverages throughout the trip and avoid alcohol and salty snacks.

If you take a few easy precautions, you can have many years of rewarding trips ahead.

What You Can Do: Make sure you take along two duplicate sets of your prescription drugs. Carry one set in your carry-on bag, and a second in your luggage, so you'll have a spare set in the event one of your bags is lost. Also, don't forget the copy of your EKG (see page 74).

#48

Consider Getting a Pet

You may not think of getting a dog or a cat in the same way you do as filling a prescription for cardiac drugs, but the right pet can offer a wealth of heart-healthy benefits.

Perhaps you owned a dog as a child, and delighted in frolicking with your pet. Upon becoming an adult, you put such joys aside as childish. If that is the case, think again.

Numerous studies have shown that pets can benefit people in a number of heart-healthy ways. Studies have shown that pet owners were more likely to survive for at least a year after being discharged from a coronary care unit. Studies have shown that playing with pets can reduce stress, lower high blood pressure, and even result in a reduction in minor health complaints. Studies have also shown having a pet can help overcome depression. Experts believe this is because of the unconditional love and acceptance that animals offer their owners. If you live alone, even a canary or parakeet can be a welcome companion.

If you need to get more exercise, again, think pets.

Owning a dog can be a great incentive for taking that daily walk. Not only does your dog expect it, but you get companionship as well.

If you're considering a pet, here are some things to keep in mind:

- Training a puppy can be an arduous task. You may prefer to skip the rambunctious puppy years in favor of an older dog. You'll be doing that dog a great favor, as puppies are often adopted, but lovely, older dogs languish in animal shelters. This is true for kittens as well.
- Some organizations sponsor programs in which pets are provided free, especially for senior citizens.
- If you live in an apartment or senior citizen residence, make sure that pets are allowed. There is nothing more heartbreaking than having to give up your pet.
- Consider your living arrangements. If you have the room, and prefer a large dog, go ahead. If you live in an apartment, remember, a toy poodle can be as bighearted as a German shepherd. Consider a mixed-breed dog as well.
- Even if you want a pure-bred dog, don't overlook dog shelters. You would be surprised at how many pure-bred dogs, some even with pedigrees, end up in a shelter, because their owners may have moved or had to give them up for another reason.
- If you're certain a pet is for you, and you have the means to care for it, don't let comments of others deter you. People who don't understand the joy of pet ownership themselves may raise their eyebrows and infer you are in a second childhood. Ignore them—it's probably just pet envy!

What You Can Do: If you are considering a dog or cat, read up on their temperaments. If you do adopt a pet, remember, it can take up to a month or so for both of you to learn to accommodate each other. Like any new relationship, give it time. The results can be very rewarding.

#49

JOIN A SUPPORT GROUP

These days, there seem to be support groups for everyone. Whether you're a compulsive eater, shopper, or talker, you can probably find your own support group. But there may be no more important a group than the support group you join for the health of your heart.

Across the country, there are thousands of cardiac support groups, or "heart clubs" awaiting you. In some cases, they may be affiliated with a cardiac rehabilitation program, but you do not necessarily have to be enrolled in the formal rehab program to join. They may be held in a local hospital, but you do not necessarily have to be a former patient.

Such groups have widely varying activities. Often, the topics deal with heart care and lifestyle changes. Local cardiologists, health authors, and dietitians may give talks on their areas of expertise. One group we visited was hosting a cardiologist, who displayed the instruments used in cardiac procedures. Another week, cardiovascular medication was the topic. But another visitor turned out to be a wildlife expert, who'd brought along some caged animals to share.

Support groups can vary a lot in character. Some groups are more serious, and offer lectures, while others are more social, and might schedule a "heart-healthy" Christmas dinner at a local restaurant. And some groups are a mixture of both.

You may want to visit several such groups before you find one where you feel you belong. Groups can differ according to their members, and you may need to find the right personality mix. Experiment. You will find yourself richly rewarded with a new set of friends, people who know what you're going through, and value your experience as well.

What You Can Do: Ask your doctor, your local hospital, or your local affiliate of the American Heart Association for the locations of heart clubs near you. Then visit a few to find the right group for you.

#50

VOLUNTEER

There's a great deal to be said for that old adage, "Helping others makes it harder to dwell on your own troubles." You can gain great satisfaction from becoming a volunteer, and help others in the process as well.

People become volunteers for all sorts of reasons. You may be a recent retiree, and find yourself bored. Your job may provide you with a paycheck, but not emotional satisfaction. You may be contemplating a job change, and want to sample a new career. Or you may want to meet new people. You may shy away from volunteering because you are afraid you don't have any skills. Just being able to greet people on the telephone with a warm, friendly voice is a skill. So is addressing envelopes, transporting an elderly person, or cuddling a baby in a hospital neonatal ward.

Do you crave culture? Many regional theater and music groups are delighted to provide free tickets to people in exchange for ushering. Do you want to work with children? Many school systems, strapped for funds, are delighted to have volunteers offer their expertise everywhere from the arts and crafts room to the school library. Some hospitals have even started programs where people can purchase "credit" toward future medical costs by volunteering!

Although you may not realize it, one area in which you have plenty of expertise is heart disease. After all, you've not only experienced heart disease, but hopefully, you've made positive changes in your lifestyle as well. Sharing your experience with others can provide them with inspiration as well as give you the determination to keep up your gains. Patients about to undergo heart surgery are often starved for personal contact. They get medical information from their doctor, but they want to draw encouragement from your first-hand experience. Mended Hearts, an organization with over four hundred local chapters, specifically provides this service to people. You could be a part of this.

The American Heart Association, for example, is eager to put your experience to good use. You can work on local campaigns, such as American Heart's Food Festival, American Heart Month, and Stroke Awareness Month. If you like to work with young people, the association sponsors many school programs as well. For addresses of both the national offices of the Heart Association and Mended Hearts, check the "Resources" section.

The important thing is to give of yourself. In doing so, you truly can forget your own problems, widen your perspectives, and meet other wonderful people doing just what you're doing.

What You Can Do: Contact your local affiliate of the American Heart Association, Mended Hearts, or check your local church, community bulletin board, or newspaper, to find other worthwhile volunteer opportunities which interest you.

Recommended Reading
and Resources

Here are some books, support groups, and other resources which you may find useful in learning more about your heart.

Books and Pamphlets

Cardiovascular Drugs

The Coronary Club. *Pocket Guide to Cardiac Drugs*, Cleveland: A Heartline Publication, 1994. (For information, see the Coronary Club. The address is listed under "Associations.")

Choosing a Doctor and Hospital

In addition to talking with your doctor, friends, or medical professionals you know, you may decide to seek some objective sources of information. Check your local library for these resources:

Sunshine, Linda, and John W. Wright. *The Best Hospitals in America*, New York: Avon, 1989.

The Cleveland Clinic Foundation has produced a series of informative guides on choosing a doctor and hospital for heart disease problems, such as:
The U.S. News and World Report Annual Guide to America's Best Hospitals, vol. 117, no. 3 (1994).

How to Choose a Doctor and Hospital. . . . If You Have Coronary Artery Disease, The Cleveland Clinic Foundation. These free pamphlets can be ordered by calling 216-444-8919 in Cleveland or 1-800-545-7718.

Cookbooks and Nutrition

The federal government offers useful information on diet, nutrition, and exercise free or at very low cost. For a free catalog, write Consumer Information Catalog, Pueblo, CO, 81109. Some examples of the publications available include *Dietary Guidelines and Your Diet, Nutritive Value of Foods*, and *Good Sources of Nutrients*.

The Coronary Club at the Cleveland Clinic Foundation offers cookbooks and videos, together or separately. They are *A Fare for the Heart* and *A Fare that Fits*. For information on ordering, contact the Coronary Club, which is listed under "Associations."

The American Heart Association Cook Book, 5th Edition, New York: Times Books, 1991.

The American Heart Association Low-Fat, Low-Cholesterol Cookbook, Scott Grundy and Mary Winston, editors. New York: Times Books, 1989.

Chiavetta, J. M., C. Barrett, and S. V. Chiavetta. *Eat, Drink and Be Healthy, A Guide to Healthful Eating and Weight Control*, North Carolina: Piedmont Publishers, 1993.

CONNOR, SONJA J., AND WILLIAM E. CONNOR. *The New American Diet System*, New York: Simon and Schuster, 1992.

GRIFFIN, GLEN, AND WILLIAM CASTELLI, M.D. *Good Fat, Bad Fat: How to Lower Your Cholesterol and Beat the Odds of a Heart Attack*, Tuscon, AZ: Fisher, 1989.

KWITEROVICH, PETER. *Beyond Cholesterol*, Los Angeles: Knightsbridge Publishers, 1991.

ORNISH, DEAN, M.D. *Eat More, Weigh Less: Dr. Dean Ornish's Life Choice Program for Losing Weight Safely While Eating Abundantly*, New York: HarperCollins, 1994.

PISCATELLA, JOSEPH C. *Controlling Your Fat Tooth*, New York: Workman, 1991.

PISCATELLA, JOSEPH C. *The Fat Tooth Fat Gram Counter* and *The Fat Tooth Restaurant and Fast Food Gram Counter*, New York: Workman, 1993.

PISCATELLA, JOSEPH, AND BERNIE PISCATELLA. *Don't Eat Your Heart Out Cookbook*, Boston: GK Hall, 1989.

PURDY, SUSAN G. *Have Your Cake and Eat It Too*, New York: William Morrow, 1993.

DIABETES

BERNSTEIN, RICHARD K., M.D. *Diabetes, Type II: Living a Long, Healthy Life Through Blood Sugar Normalization*, New York: Prentice Hall Press, 1990.

FITNESS

LAWRENCE, RONALD M., AND SANDRA ROSENZWEIG. *Going the Distance: The Right Way to Exercise for People Over 40*, Los Angeles: Jeremy P. Tarcher, 1987.

FLETCHER, BARBARA J., *Exercise for Heart and Health*, Atlanta: Pritchett & Hull, 1993.

Family Relationships

Levin, Rhonda F. *Heartmates: A Survival Guide for the Cardiac Spouse*, Fort Wayne, IN: P.B. Co., 1990.

Sotile, Wayne M., ph.d. *Heart Illness and Intimacy: How Caring Relationships Aid Recovery*, Baltimore: Johns Hopkins University Press, 1992.

Health Care Issues

Barrett, Stephen, m.d., and the Editors of Consumer Reports. *Health Schemes, Scams and Frauds*, Mount Vernon, NY: Consumer Reports Books, Consumers Union, 1990.

Inlander, Charles B., and Ed Weiner. *Take This Book to the Hospital with You: A Consumer Guide to Surviving Your Hospital Stay*, New York: Pantheon, 1991.

McCann, Karen Keating. *Take Charge of Your Hospital Stay: A "Start Smart" Guide for Patients and Care Partners*, New York: Plenum, 1994.

Hogue, Kathleen, Cheryl Jensen, and Kathleen McClurg Urban. *The Complete Guide to Health Insurance*, New York: Avon, 1990.

Stutz, David R., m.d., Bernard Feder, ph.d., and the Editors of Consumer Reports. *The Savvy Patient: How to Be an Active Participant in Your Medical Care*, Mount Vernon, NY: Consumer Reports Books, Consumers Union, 1990.

Heart Disease

Budnick, Herbert N., ph.d., and Scott Robert Hays. *Heart to Heart: A Guide to the Psychological Aspects of Heart Disease*, Santa Fe, NM: HealthPress, 1991.

Hellerstein, Herman, m.d., and Paul Perry. *Healing Your Heart*, New York: Simon and Schuster, 1991.

Kowalski, Robert E., *Eight Steps to a Healthy Heart: The*

Complete Guide to Heart Disease Prevention and Recovery from Heart Attack and Bypass Surgery, New York: Warner Books Inc., 1994.

KWITEROVICH, PETER. *The Johns Hopkins Complete Guide for Preventing and Reversing Heart Disease*, Roseville, CA: Prima, 1993.

HEART DISEASE (WOMEN)

PASHKOW, FREDRIC J., M.D., AND CHARLOTTE LIBOV. *The Woman's Heart Book: The Complete Guide to Keeping a Healthy Heart and What to Do If Things Go Wrong*, New York: Plume, 1994.

The Healthy Heart Handbook for Women, Washington: National Institutes of Health, 1989.

MENOPAUSE AND HORMONE REPLACEMENT THERAPY

The use of hormone replacement therapy is controversial and not all the authors of these books agree. Reading differing viewpoints will give you the information you need to make an individual decision based on your medical evaluation, your doctor's recommendation, and your individual wishes.

GILLESPIE, CLARK. *Hormones, Hot Flashes and Mood Swings: Living Through the Ups and Downs of Menopause*, New York: Perennial Library, 1989.

NACHTIGALL, LILA, M.D., AND JOAN RATTNER HEILMAN. *Estrogen: The Facts Can Change Your Life*, New York: HarperCollins, 1991.

NOTELOVITZ, MORRIS, M.D., AND DIANA TONNESSEN. *Menopause and Midlife Health*, New York: St. Martin's, 1993.

RINZLER, CAROL ANN. *Estrogen and Breast Cancer: A Warning to Women*, New York: MacMillan, 1993.

SACHS, JUDITH. *What Women Should Know About Menopause*, New York: Dell, 1991.

UTIAN, WULF H., AND RUTH S. JACOBOWITZ. *Managing Your Menopause*, New York: Prentice Hall Press, 1990.

SEXUALITY

BERNIE ZILBERGELD. *The New Male Sexuality*, New York: Bantam, 1992.

HEIMAN, JULIA, AND JOSEPH LOPICCOLO. *Becoming Orgasmic: A Sexual Growth Program for Women*, New York: Prentice Hall, 1988.

STRESS REDUCTION

DAVIS, M., E. R. ESHELMAN, AND M. MCKAY. *The Relaxation and Stress Reduction Workbook*, 3rd Edition, Oakland, CA: New Harbinger, 1988.

STROKE

AMERICAN HEART ASSOCIATION. *Family Guide to Stroke*, New York: Times Books, 1994.

SURGERY & RECUPERATION (GENERAL)

COHAN, CAROL, M.A., JUNE B. PIMM, PH.D., AND JAMES R. JUDE, M.D. *A Patient's Guide to Heart Surgery: Understanding the Practical and Emotional Aspects of Heart Surgery*, New York: HarperCollins, 1991.

WOMEN'S HEALTH CARE (GENERAL)

SHEPHARD, BRUCE D., M.D., F.A.C.O.B., AND CARROLL A. SHEPHARD, R.N., PH.D. *The Complete Guide to Women's Health*, 2nd Edition, New York: Penguin, 1990.

WHITE, EVELYN C. *The Black Women's Health Book: Speaking for Ourselves*, Seattle, WA: The Seal Press, 1990.

WOLFE, SIDNEY M., M.D. AND THE PUBLIC CITIZEN HEALTH RESEARCH GROUP WITH RHONDA DONKIN JONES. *Women's*

Health Alert, Reading, Massachusetts: Addison-Wesley Publishing Group, Inc., 1991.

NEWSLETTERS

Newsletters written for the general public about health topics are becoming increasingly popular. Here is a roundup of particularly useful ones. Since prices may change, check before ordering.

Heartline

Award-winning monthly newsletter designed for heart patients and others interested in their cardiovascular health. Edited by Dr. Fredric J. Pashkow, it is published with the active support of the Cleveland Clinic Foundation. $24 per year. For more information, contact the Coronary Club, which is listed under "Associations."

Harvard Heart Letter

A monthly newsletter published by the Harvard Medical School Health Publication Group which discusses heart-related topics in depth. $30 per year. Harvard Heart Letter, P.O. Box 420234, Palm Court, FL 32142-0234.

Cardiac Alert

Published monthly for the purpose of educating for the prevention of heart disease. Edited by Dr. Jorge C. Rios, George Washington University Medical Center. $75 per year. Phillips Publishing, Inc., 7811 Montrose Road, Potomac, MD 20854.

Medical Abstracts Newsletter

A monthly roundup of news on medical topics in general (not only cardiology) written in interesting, easy to understand language. Includes full citations so readers can look up interesting journal articles themselves. $24.95 per year. Medical Abstracts Newsletter, Box 2170, Teaneck, NJ 07666.

Diet-Heart Newsletter

Published quarterly by health-book author Robert Kowalksi,

offers nutritional information, recipes and tips. $18 per year. Diet-Heart Newsletter, P.O. Box 2039, Venice, CA 90294.

ASSOCIATIONS AND SUPPORT GROUPS

Many hospitals have support groups for heart patients, which offer activities ranging from educational to social events. Bear in mind that you do not necessarily have to have been treated at that hospital to join. For information, contact your local hospital, or these organizations:

American Heart Association
Consult your telephone book for the local chapter or contact the national organization at 7320 Greenville Avenue, Dallas, TX 75231.

The Coronary Club
This organization offers answers to questions, discounts on products and services of interest to members, and books, videotapes, and other materials by mail order. It is the publisher of *Heartline* (see page 181, under "Newsletters"). For more information, contact the Coronary Club, Inc., 9500 Euclid Ave., EE-37, Cleveland, OH 44195. Telephone: 800-478-4255.

Mended Hearts
7320 Greenville Avenue
Dallas, TX 75231

The American Cancer Society
Consult your telephone book for your local chapter, or contact the national headquarters at 1599 Clifton Road, N.E., Atlanta, GA 30329-4251

INDEX

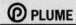

℗ PLUME

ISSUES IN HEALTH AND MEDICINE